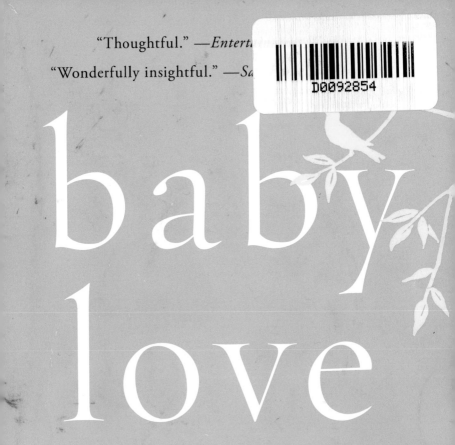

"Thoughtful." —*Enterta*

"Wonderfully insightful." —*Sa*

D0092854

baby
love

CHOOSING MOTHERHOOD

AFTER

A LIFETIME *of* AMBIVALENCE

REBECCA
WALKER

AUTHOR OF THE NATIONAL BESTSELLER *BLACK, WHITE, AND JEWISH*

Praise for *Baby Love*

"A thoughtful and amusing play-by-play of pregnancy and birth, investigating the difference between the theory surrounding motherhood and the scary, messy, snuggly practice of it."
—*The Washington Post Book World*

"Walker . . . uses her sharp intelligence to examine the joyful, terrifying ride to parenthood and the complex roles of mother and child. As Walker, now thirty-seven, begins her pregnancy in 2004, she is torn between the desire to be a loving daughter—to a brilliant, difficult woman who has her own ambivalence about motherhood—and the desire to love unconditionally as a mom. . . . You know she'll do just fine embracing motherhood, in all its sloppy, intimate selflessness and glory." —*People* (3½ stars)

"[A] wonderfully insightful writer . . . offers an unflinching look at her doubts, her anxieties, even her pride in knowing she's joined a special club as her pregnancy begins to show. And she offers a realistic account of labor and delivery . . . Tells a poignant love story of herself and her son." —The Associated Press

"[A] powerful new memoir . . . Walker's story is accessible and richly textured, told with humor, wit and warmth." —*Publishers Weekly*

"Walker, a prominent feminist and author of *Black, White, and Jewish,* deconstructs the struggle of many women who, though weaned on the idea of a woman's right to choice, have viewed motherhood 'with more than a little suspicion.' " —*Entertainment Weekly*

"A poignant love story of herself and her son."
—*San Francisco Chronicle*

continued . . .

"Third-wave feminist Walker, the daughter of author Alice Walker and a bestselling scribe in her own right, continues chronicling her life with this journal of her decision to become a mother in her midthirties." —*Library Journal*

"Walker sways on a kind of scary, sublime suspension bridge, stretched between being somebody's child and becoming somebody's mother, and turning her fiercely compassionate intelligence to both. Thanks to her unique vision, the familiar views along the way become nothing short of astounding." —Catherine Newman, author of *Waiting for Birdy*

"[Written] with honesty, passion, intelligence, wisdom, and insight . . . *Baby Love* will resonate with any woman who has fallen in love with her baby or is wrestling with choosing motherhood." —Miriam Arond, Editor in Chief of *Child* magazine

"*Baby Love* is a gorgeous memoir, confessional in the most universal of ways. In richly detailed prose, Walker takes us on her journey toward motherhood, and womanhood, and, ultimately, personhood, with unflinching honesty and raw, painfully beautiful storytelling." —Alisa Valdes-Rodriguez, author of *Make Him Look Good*

Praise for *Black, White, and Jewish*

"Compelling."
—*The Washington Post*

"A complex, all-American story."
—*USA Today*

"Walker skillfully depicts her tangled upbringing, full of disappointment and privilege."
—*Time*

"Walker masterfully illuminates differences between black and white America. . . . A heartbreaking tale of self-creation." —*People*

"A cautionary tale about the power of race in shaping identity . . . A highly readable debut."
—*Entertainment Weekly*

"A well-written refusal to ignore old wounds." —*The Boston Globe*

"Her outsider status equips her with a sharp eye for analysis and narrative detail. And her restrained prose is refreshing in this age of gushing confession."
—*The Washington Post Book World*

"*Black, White, and Jewish* is a frank, detail-rich look at her upbringing."
—*Chicago Tribune*

"Her book is an attempt to not only come to grips with her own identity, but to expose the pain and turmoil that come with shifting back and forth. . . . It is a stunningly honest account, almost painfully self-revelatory."
—*San Francisco Chronicle*

"A poignant, spare memoir."
—*Chicago Sun-Times*

"*Black, White, and Jewish* is Rebecca Walker's anthem of independence, the compelling diary of a 'Movement Baby' who combats her own racial insecurities."
—*The Dallas Morning News*

ALSO BY REBECCA WALKER

To Be Real: Telling the Truth and
Changing the Face of Feminism

Black, White, and Jewish:
Autobiography of a Shifting Self

What Makes a Man:
22 Writers Imagine the Future

BABY LOVE

CHOOSING MOTHERHOOD
After a Lifetime of Ambivalence

Rebecca Walker

RIVERHEAD BOOKS

New York

RIVERHEAD BOOKS
Published by the Penguin Group
Penguin Group (USA) Inc.
375 Hudson Street, New York, New York 10014, USA

Penguin Group (Canada), 90 Eglinton Avenue East, Suite 700, Toronto, Ontario M4P 2Y3,
Canada (a division of Pearson Penguin Canada Inc.) • Penguin Books Ltd., 80 Strand,
London WC2R 0RL, England • Penguin Group Ireland, 25 St. Stephen's Green, Dublin 2,
Ireland (a division of Penguin Books Ltd.) • Penguin Group (Australia), 250 Camberwell Road,
Camberwell, Victoria 3124, Australia (a division of Pearson Australia Group Pty. Ltd.) •
Penguin Books India Pvt. Ltd., 11 Community Centre, Panchsheel Park, New Delhi—110 017,
India • Penguin Group (NZ), 67 Apollo Drive, Rosedale, North Shore 0632, New Zealand
(a division of Pearson New Zealand Ltd.) • Penguin Books (South Africa) (Pty.) Ltd.,
24 Sturdee Avenue, Rosebank, Johannesburg 2196, South Africa

Penguin Books Ltd., Registered Offices: 80 Strand, London WC2R 0RL, England

The publisher does not have any control over and does not assume any responsibility
for author or third-party websites or their content.

Copyright © 2007 by Rebecca Walker
Cover design © 2007 Gabriele Wilson
Book design by Amanda Dewey

The passages on pages 11, 79, and 147 are quoted from the Baby Centre website
(www.babycentre.co.uk).

All rights reserved.
No part of this book may be reproduced, scanned, or distributed in any printed or electronic form
without permission. Please do not participate in or encourage piracy of copyrighted materials in
violation of the author's rights. Purchase only authorized editions.
RIVERHEAD is a registered trademark of Penguin Group (USA) Inc.
The RIVERHEAD logo is a trademark of Penguin Group (USA) Inc.

First Riverhead hardcover edition: March 2007
First Riverhead trade paperback edition: March 2008
Riverhead trade paperback ISBN: 978-1-59448-288-5

The Library of Congress has catalogued the Riverhead hardcover edition as follows:

Walker, Rebecca, date.
Baby love : choosing motherhood after
a lifetime of ambivalence / Rebecca Walker.
p.   cm.
ISBN 978-1-59448-943-3
1. Walker, Rebecca.   2. Pregnant women—United States—Biography.   3. Pregnancy—
Psychological aspects.   4. Motherhood—Psychological aspects.   5. Ambivalence   I. Title.
RG560.W35 2007   2006037160
618.2'00[B]92—dc22

PRINTED IN THE UNITED STATES OF AMERICA

10 9 8 7 6 5 4 3 2 1

For Tenzin,
who made it real

April 8

I'm pregnant.

I just got off the phone with the nurse from Dr. Lowen's office. I picked up the old brown Trimline phone that's been in this retreat cabin of my mother's forever, and a woman's voice asked for me and I said, This is she, and the voice said, It's Becky from Dr. Lowen's office. And I said, Uh-huh. Then Becky said, The result from the latest test was positive, and I said, Positive? And she said, Yes, you are no longer borderline pregnant.

No longer borderline pregnant? I thought I might fall over. I looked out the window at the leaves of the poplar trees shimmering in the breeze. My eyes settled on a vulture falling from the sky in a perfect spiral. He was flapping then gliding, flapping then gliding as he descended, and I thought to myself: I will remember this moment and that vulture for the rest of my life. I thought to myself: That vulture is a sign. A part of me is dying.

And then the nurse said, Hello? And I said, Yes, I am here. Are you sure I am pregnant? And she said, Yes. And I said, Really? You're not going to call me back in two hours and say you made a mistake? She said, No. And I said, Well, how do you know? She sighed. It was a ridiculous question, but since she had been telling me for a week that after three blood draws they still couldn't tell if I was really pregnant, I felt justified. So I pushed. What do you know today that you didn't yesterday? And she said, The HCG levels are definitely going up. HCG levels? Yes, in the last twenty-four hours the pregnancy hormone count has risen from 700 to over 2,300, and that usually means a healthy, robust beginning.

And then I had what could only be the first twinges of the maternal instinct. Healthy and robust? A huge smile spread across my face. That's my baby! And then it was as if the synapses in my brain sending exploratory signals to my uterus finally made contact. Aye, mate, is it a go down there? Yes, yes, Captain, we're full steam ahead!

I was convinced that getting off the phone would exponentially increase my chances of reverting to not-pregnant, but I released Becky anyway and stumbled over to the bathroom, where Glen, my life partner and father of our soon-to-be-born baby, was shaving. I looked into his eyes and tried to keep myself from screaming and jumping up and down. We did it, I said. He grinned. Well, I guess that puts the whole motility question to rest. And I said, I guess it does. Then I wrapped my arms around him and buried my face in his chest, and he wrapped his arms around me and rested his chin on the top of my head.

I was in ecstatic bliss for about ninety seconds, and then it hit me: an avalanche of dread that took my breath away. Pregnant?

A baby? What have I done? I looked at Glen. He was going through his own reality check, which brought me even closer to the brink of total hysteria. But then, before I could burst into tears and run screaming out of the room, he pulled me into his arms. You are going to be a fantastic mother, he said to me, to my fear. His love overwhelmed me, and I started to cry big, wet tears onto his favorite black shirt.

We're going to have a baby.

One

FOR THE LAST FIFTEEN YEARS I have told everyone—friends, family, hairdressers, editors, cabdrivers, doctors, and anyone else who would listen—that I wanted a baby. *I want to have a baby,* I would say with urgency or a wistful longing, or both. And I meant what I said, I really did, I just had no idea what I was talking about. I had almost no actual experience of babies, so the object of my wanting was abstract, the display of it ritualized. *I want to have a baby* was something I said, a statement that evoked a trajectory, a general direction for my life.

The truth is, I was wracked with ambivalence. I had the usual questions: When, with whom, and how the hell was I going to afford it? But there was something else, too, a question common—if not always conscious—to women of my generation, women raised to view motherhood with more than a little suspicion. Can I survive having a baby? Will I lose myself—my body, my mind, my *options*—and be left trapped, resentful, and irretrievably overwhelmed? If I have a baby, we wonder silently to ourselves, will I die?

To compound matters, I had a tempestuous relationship with my mother, and feared the inevitable kickback sure to follow such a final and dramatic departure from daughterhood. What if, instead of joy and excitement, my mother felt threatened by the baby, and pushed even further into the margins of my life? What if, then, out of jealousy and her own discontent, she launched covert or not-so-covert strikes against my irrefutable separateness, now symbolized so completely by becoming a mother myself?

Because mothers make us, because they map our emotional terrain before we even know we are capable of having an emotional terrain, they know just where to stick the dynamite. With a few small power plays—a skeptical comment, the withholding of approval or praise—a mother can devastate a daughter. Decades of subtle undermining can stunt a daughter, or so monopolize her energy that she in effect stunts herself. Muted, fearful, riddled with self-doubt, she can remain trapped in daughterhood forever, the one place she feels confident she knows the rules.

I was not the only daughter in a dyad of this kind. When I looked around, I saw them everywhere: in my extended family, at my lectures on college campuses, on line at Target, on their own show on TV. Childless and codependent, the daughter did some macabre human version of dying on the vine. The mother kept the reality of her own mortality at bay by thwarting her daughter's every attempt to psychologically leave the nest.

It seemed that these mothers did not realize that they had to *give* adulthood to their daughters by stepping down, stepping back, stepping away, and letting the daughter take center stage. These mothers did not seem to know, with all their potions and philosophies, their desires to rehabilitate ancient scripts of gender and identity, that there is a natural order, and that natural order involves passing the scepter to offspring with unconditional love and pride.

Or pay the price.

BECAUSE AS A WRITER I do my best research in the lives of others, at least once a week I sat conversing—over tea, on subway platforms, at the farmers' market, in ornate, fancy hotel lobbies—about motherhood with women who either had done the deed and lived to tell, or who were surveying the same terrain of possibility.

I spoke to single moms and partnered moms, and moms who lost their children to disease. I spoke to stay-at-home moms, working moms, CEO moms, moms on welfare. One mom I met conceived through in vitro fertilization at age forty-five. Another orchestrated different sperm donors over several pregnancies. One "got pregnant" at eighteen and spent the rest of her life trying to recover. I spent an afternoon talking with a poor mom who relied on faith to provide for her sixth child on the way. I spent several years talking to middle-class moms who couldn't figure out how to support the two kids they already had.

I talked to men, too, about the joys and risks of parenthood, but my time with them was different. It wasn't punctuated with anecdotes, or even held together by narrative. Men explored the topic of my pregnancy with meaningful glances and gentle touches of assurance to the small of my back. They encouraged me with knowing nods and unwavering attention, sometimes silently offering themselves, other times letting me know they wished it could be them.

Women gave me narrative and men gave me alchemy, their approbation running like a current into my womb.

My life was full of these elucidating encounters, but strangely, none of them seemed to bring me any closer to what I said I wanted. Unconsciously, I longed to give birth to a child. Consciously, I managed the risk of actually having one by viewing it as one option among many, a wonderful possibility to peruse at will. Like choosing which coast to live on or what apartment to take, I would consider potential outcomes and make my best, informed decision.

Because I am a woman of privilege, a product of the women's movement, and a student of cultural relativism, I believed that neither choice would be inherently better than the other. Each had pluses and minuses, and so it would not be the choice itself, but how I interpreted the choice that would make the difference. Los Angeles or New York? High floor or great location? To baby or not to baby?

Ultimately, it was like trying to steer a boat with a banana. I had no idea what was going on, no clue whatsoever. I didn't know that I was already in the water, that the tide was coming in fast, and that I had no option other than to be taken out to sea. I didn't know that the longing, fear, and ambivalence were part of the pregnancy, the birth, and everything that came after. I didn't know that the showdown between the ideas of my mother's gen-

You may not look pregnant at this point but your embryo's heart, no bigger than a poppyseed, has already begun to beat and pump blood. . . . The embryo itself is about a quarter of an inch long and looks more like a tadpole than a human.

April 10

I called my mother last night to tell her the news, because I promised she would be the first to know. When I told her I have never been happier, she was quiet. She said she was shocked, which was shocking to me since I've been telling her for a year that all I want is to write books and have babies. When we were about to hang up, she asked me to check her garden. I said okay and told her that I had ordered some outdoor lights for this tiny house she lets me use, and that the new tile in the shower is almost finished. Then I hung up and started to cry.

I don't know if I wanted her to be like all the other mothers I've seen get the news, whooping for joy and crying and jumping up and down, but when she didn't, I was overcome with doubt. Flopping down on the bed, I regressed all the way back to high school, when I got my acceptance letter from Yale. I was ecstatic, and proudly presented the letter to my mother as she cooked dinner. She calmly husked a few ears of corn, and then asked why I would want to go to a conservative bastion of male privilege. It didn't take ten seconds for me to question my own dreams. Why *did* I want to go to one of the most well-respected colleges in the world?

Why *am* I having a baby?

Glen found me lying on the floor, practically catatonic, staring out into space with tears streaming down my face. We talked for a long time about rites of passage, and how everyone is bound to have a reaction that has nothing to do with me. Mothers and fathers have to reckon with their own mortality, with becoming grandparents, and what that means about where they are in the life cycle. He told me to get ready, people say the strangest things when you tell them you are pregnant because it brings up so much for them.

Like I did when I met with my literary agent about this book. She told me she was pregnant with her third baby, and I said something awful like, How can you possibly take care of three children? Or even worse, Was it an accident? Then I grilled her on whether she would be able to take care of her baby, my book, and me. I was seized with anxiety in the moment, but really, her pregnancy rang my bell. Happy, vibrant, strong, direct. I thought, If she can be a VP of her company, gaze adoringly at a photo of her husband whipped out of her purse, and talk about how her kids are the greatest gifts of her life, this baby thing must be possible.

I went to sleep pondering whether I got more positive messaging about having a baby from my agent in thirty-five minutes than I did from my mother in thirty-five years.

April 13

I'm back in Berkeley, in my apartment that suddenly looks like a broom closet. Where am I going to put a crib?

Dr. Lowen ordered an ultrasound this morning to make sure that there really is a baby growing inside me. Isn't that why I'd asked Becky ten times if she was sure? Dr. Lowen says we need to know that the fetus is inside my uterus and not ectopic. *Ectopic!* Glen had to calm me down. All I could think was that a problem must have showed up on the last blood test and Dr. Lowen didn't want to tell me on the phone and give me heart failure.

Glen drove me to the hospital, and then tried to distract me in the waiting room with bad jokes and blueberries. I kept asking him what we'd do if the baby were ectopic, if I lost the baby before I even had her. How is it possible to feel so attached so soon? By the time the technician called my name, I was sure it was all going to end in tragedy. She poked and rubbed and scanned and prodded my uterus for about twenty minutes, looking for the tiny cluster of cells and shaking her head until I was convinced the whole thing was a fluke. At that exact moment, when I squeezed Glen's hand and said, Well, maybe we don't have a baby after all, the technician pushed the button on her mouse ball and drew a line from one point to the other. Got it.

So now it's super-duper official. I've got a baby growing in my uterus. It's really the most surreal, ridiculous, amazing thing.

April 15

Rushed around, getting ready to fly to Minneapolis to speak on the importance of mentorship in young women's lives at the Minnesota Conference on Adolescent Females. Usually I like going to Minneapolis, but today I am just so tired. I can't imagine getting on a plane and then turning around the next day to come back. It's only three and a half hours each way, but at the moment, Minnesota may as well be the North Pole.

I was up all night consumed with anxiety about money—mine and every other mother's. By most standards I am well off, but now that all I do is think about the stuff I am going to have to pay for, like the college education that's going to cost two million dollars in eighteen years, I don't know. I remember my mother making endless calculations on brown paper bags and blank pages in her journal when I was a child, and my father sitting at the dining-room table writing checks out every month, his brow furrowed and intense. They must have felt the same way, going over the numbers again and again, wondering how it was all going to work out.

I woke up feeling guilty for even thinking about all this. Most people in the world raise their children with far less than I have. But that's the thing, isn't it? Even when you have enough money to pay for nonessentials like organic produce and designer toothpaste, there is still the yawning fear of not having, losing everything, living in deprivation.

I definitely thought about money long before this baby moved into my womb. I worried about how we were going to send my ex-girlfriend's son, Solomon, to boarding school. I worried about the cost of health insurance, and how little money I put into my IRA. But now my thinking has a frightening urgency. I find myself wondering how all the other pregnant women and mothers and fathers manage what basically boils down to sheer terror in the face of so much responsibility. Religion suddenly makes a lot more sense. So does workaholism. And Xanax. And back-to-the-land movements that emphasize doing more with less.

I bolted out of bed this morning to research the Voluntary Simplicity movement. I read dozens of entries by people named Sinnan and Marigold who grow their own food, wear only three pairs of pants, and make their own soap. I learned that an American baby consumes two hundred times more of the earth's resources than a baby from Eritrea.

By the time Glen woke up, I was deep in my closet, figuring out how many pairs of shoes and sweaters I could transform into fossil fuel in order to justify having an American baby. When he asked what I was doing, I snapped that I was freaking out about money, wasn't that obvious? He sat in the big chair in our bedroom and put his feet up, watching me. I mean really, I said, how are we going to put this baby through college?

He paused. There are always student loans. Student loans? I said, lifting my head out of a storage bin at the back of the closet. I had forgotten about those. Weren't several of my friends still paying off their student loans, and didn't they seem as neurotic and happy as anybody else? I gently extracted a purple sweater from the giveaway pile.

Having a partner who thinks rationally and optimistically even
when I cannot does not eliminate my anxiety about supporting
another human being for the next twenty years, but it certainly
helps.

April 22

I made it back from Minneapolis last night in one piece, but
this morning I almost killed myself with a spritz of perfume. I've
been trying to ignore the growing intensity of my reaction to
smells, but today I just couldn't. I took off all my clothes, got
back in the shower, and scrubbed off the barest hint of perfume I
had put on my neck. Then I drove to my homeopath's office
grumbling about what a bummer it is that I can't wear scent
without feeling like I am on a capsizing catamaran.

Marie's excitement cheered me up. I feel it's her victory, too,
because from the moment I said I wanted to have a baby, she's
been right there with me, giving me flower tinctures and vitamin
D, progesterone tablets and visualizations of myself big and
pregnant with a happy, healthy baby.

After the hugs and whoops, I confessed that I almost gave up
on our noninvasive plan because I thought that after six months,
I wasn't getting any younger and should try the medical model. I
told her that I had already scheduled the HSG (hysterosalpin-
gogram), where they inject dye into your fallopian tubes to see if
they work, and I had a prescription for the ovulation-inducing
Clomid in my bag. It was the preliminary, precautionary pregnancy test Dr. Lowen ordered that revealed the fruit of our homeopathic work.

Marie didn't bat an eye or get judgmental, and that's why I love her, my kindhearted M.D. homeopath. She just said, Well, good thing you didn't have to go through all of that! and started making a list of all the foods I should start eating: farm-raised lamb, eggs, Norwegian fish oil.

Then we talked about whether I should stop taking the low-dose antidepressant I've been taking to counteract God-knows-how-many generations of depression in my family tree. The thought of quitting cold turkey is terrifying. I have gone from being skeptical of my little purple pill, to angry that I need it, to hugely grateful to all of the good people in big pharma involved in creating it. I'm not exaggerating when I say it has allowed me to have some semblance of a normal life.

As I looked on expectantly, Marie checked her big pharmaceutical handbook to see if trials have been done on pregnant women. Limited trials, she said, but the drug is rated B for pregnancy, which means it's not stellar, but it is doable. I looked at her across the desk covered with mugs, supplements, and files. Unless we know for sure that it will hurt the baby, I said, I just don't think it's a good idea for me to stop. The first thing depression takes from me is hope, and I am pretty sure I can't have a baby without that. She agreed.

I left her office feeling good about the decision, but still full of concern. In addition to all of the other ways I can lose or harm this baby, I can now add the possibility of damaging his nervous system with what to some is an optional drug.

I also wonder about straddling the medical ob/gyn and homeopathic worlds. In theory they are compatible, but in reality I am not so sure. Dr. Lowen is all business and efficiency, Formica and fluorescents, and Marie is soft lighting and colorful art, hugs and flower remedies. Of course, Marie says they are compatible—after all, she is an M.D.—and Dr. Lowen tries to sound sympathetic when I mention the natural methods. But in real life, there seems to be an eerie disconnect between the two that leaves me slightly uncertain about both.

Which brings me back to where I started, at the perfume that triggered today's initial bout of uncertainty about what may be the biggest decision I've ever made. Is this the beginning of the end? Is this the first of many things I love that I will have to give up for the baby? First perfume and then sanity, sleep, and travel to interesting places? Is this what everybody means when they say your life will never be the same? Say goodbye to emotional stability? Say goodbye to amber, lavender, rose, and sandalwood? Say goodbye to Brooklyn, Paris, and Dakar?

Is there any peace in this process? I struggled for years to decide whether to become a parent. Now that it's happening, I'm plagued by apocalyptic visions of how it's going to turn out. Has it always been this way? Is this elixir of ambivalence and anxiety the universal experience of motherhood, or is it just America, circa right now?

Two

MANY WOMEN SAY that for as long as they can remember, they've wanted to have a baby. They say that playing with dolls was their first introduction to the idea of motherhood, that they've known since childhood they would give birth.

I didn't play with dolls. I never knew, the way I knew that I would go to college and eventually earn a living, that I would have a baby. Unlike the women who can't pinpoint exactly how or why they came to the feeling, I remember exactly when and where I felt the first pang of maternal desire.

I was in Africa, in a country so foreign that none of my old thoughts about myself could hold. I found I could live without running water and electricity. I could survive armed soldiers and random searches of my bags on public buses. I could be friends, sisters even, with women who covered themselves from head to toe in swaths of black cloth.

And, because of a man I met, I could fantasize about having a child.

Ade was and still is a devout Muslim. We met in the middle of Ramadan and spent hours on the rooftop of my guesthouse talking about his culture. In conversations I dominated, I questioned him pointedly about how women were treated. What were his thoughts about the veil? Forget niceties. I wanted to know if the women in his family were circumcised. I asked these questions, but I can't say I was open to Ade's answers. Though only twenty years old, I was positive I knew much more than Ade about the gender politics of his country from the books I had read and women I had befriended.

But Ade wasn't affected by my arrogance. He listened to each of my criticisms intently, and responded with a rather (compared to mine) complex view. He told me first what he believed (women are as powerful as men and should be respected as equals), and then explained what the Quran taught (one of the Prophet's wives was a businesswoman who financed his rise), and then finally conceded the interpretation of those with power (women should be subordinate and obedient). He was adamant that there was no circumcision, but promised to ask Fatima, a rare female friend with whom he could talk about these things, and tell me what she said.

What can I say? I fell for Ade during those conversations. Ade could talk. He wasn't afraid of me. He seemed to know his own mind, to have considered the issues I raised and come to some decisions, decisions I respected even if I didn't agree. He was unfamiliar with the intellectual combat I was honing at college, and his lack of competitiveness allowed me a relaxed curiosity I had not known. When he left, I felt awake and alive, as if the door of everything I had learned had been blown open.

Because of this and other factors too numerous to mention here, I stayed several months with Ade, and one day, after I had convinced my traveling companion to go to Tanzania without me and I no longer knew when I would leave Ade's tiny island or why, I went out in a dhow with Ade and some friends. We were far from the shore, out on the open sea. I was wearing a gray T-shirt and Ade's blue-and-white-striped *kikoi* around my waist. Ade was balancing himself on the hull of the boat, releasing the rope that let the ship's battered sail unfurl in the wind.

As the boat picked up speed, I leaned back on my elbows and imagined a future with Ade. Even though his culture and beliefs ran up against everything I knew and held sacred, I found myself fantasizing that I would spend the rest of my life with him, that I would wash clothes by hand in a basin with two cups of water, and give up reading at night because we wouldn't have electricity. I dreamed that I would dress modestly and respect his mother, that I would learn to cook delicious food in huge aluminum pots over an open fire.

And then the fantasy I'd never had: the dream that was less about Ade than it was about what I suddenly saw as possible for my life. I would have a baby with Ade, two babies, three babies, as many babies as I could.

A baby. I want to have a baby.

And then, just as quickly, I turned my eyes from the sky to the floor of the old boat and thought, *That's ridiculous. I can't have a baby. I have to finish school and start my career.*

April 25

I'm back in Mendocino. The drive up from Berkeley last night was *awful*. I was so nauseated going around the curves, we had to stop the car. As I leaned out the window gulping air and smelling the blood of fresh roadkill thirty feet away, I thought seriously about walking, or going to sleep in the backseat and trying again in the morning. I was so happy to get to the gate to the house. I threw myself on the ground and lay there smelling the dirt and waiting for the world to stop spinning.

I'm nauseated and exhausted, but none of that has any effect whatsoever on my urge to nest. I'm always trying to make a home because I moved so many times as a kid, but now my nesting thing is on, like, hyperturbo overdrive. My mind just goes tick, tick, tick across every room, scanning for possible upgrades and nooks that could be softer, more comfortable, more homey.

After we unpacked the bags and bags of food, and after I set up my desk by hooking up my laptop and getting the lamp positioned just so, I checked the shower tile and the light fixtures. Then I went around and made a list of the other changes I needed to talk to Carl, my friend the builder/contractor, about.

I don't know how he does it, but Glen just reads and eats and relaxes as I run around trying to make everything perfect. By just leaving me alone, he gives me permission to be myself and I *love* that. I feel the animal aspect of it, too. I am making the nest and he's standing over it, protecting all three of us while I do it.

April 28

Today I feel sad, tired, and unsure about everything. Like I have no real support outside of Glen for having this baby. Like I have no healthy models for how to have a family. My parents barely spoke to each other for twenty-five years. After raising two children together, my father and stepmother live somewhat separate lives. My relationships thus far have been, um, educational, but not terribly successful.

I am trying not to ruminate on all of this and to believe that I can reverse the divorce dynamic by staying with Glen until one of us dies, but it's like my mind is in a vise. When I am not throwing up or wanting to throw up, I am having anxiety attacks about being homeless, unable to keep my family together, and making the same mistakes my parents made. Other variations on the doomsday theme running through my mind: miscarriage, miscarriage, and miscarriage.

I would rather die than hurt my baby, but I think I would actually die if I lost my baby.

Is that a depressed thought or a normal pregnancy feeling?

April 30

Today I was outrageously nauseated, but went looking at gates with Carl anyway. I think I can safely describe Carl as an aging hippie. He built many houses in Anderson Valley and along the Mendocino coast, and is incredibly knowledgeable about all things having to do with construction, environmental preservation, and a host of other things we haven't yet talked about. He's in his sixties, and has a little shake that makes hitting nails a challenge sometimes, but I consider it a blessing that he has agreed to help reclaim this little house of my mother's from dry rot, wasps, and a general state of dilapidation.

After finding a fairly nice gate that I will be able to open and shut without too much effort even at nine months, we went to see the house he has been building for his family for fifteen years. His wife, Martine, made me chamomile tea with honey for the nausea I told her was flattening me, and Carl brought over a book of photographs of the home birth of his second child.

The pictures were incredible. Carl was young and cute, with long, braided hippie hair and an embroidered denim shirt. In the pictures, he's rubbing his wife's back and holding her hand and kissing her. She's lying down, fully naked and fully pregnant, surrendering to the process first on her back, then on her side, then on all fours when the baby is ready to come out. The room is dim so the baby won't be shocked, and Carl's first child, Tomas, who was four or five, holds a flashlight so they can take pictures.

Martine and Carl sent me home with something called *The Birth Book,* a collection of birth stories published by a midwifery collective Carl worked with in the seventies. After reading the stories of ten or fifteen women and their partners and midwives, I feel more than ever that I want to have a home birth. I can't imagine having the baby in a hospital. I just don't see how lying flat on your back can possibly be the best way to have a baby. I mean, for starters, it works *against* gravity.

May 4

I had my first official prenatal appointment today. It was like being on a conveyor belt at the baby-making factory. I was weighed, my urine tested, and seven vials of blood were extracted from my arm. I was asked about my mother's health, my father's, sister's, and brother's. Then back to the beginning for Glen's family info. The doctor briefly skipped a rock across the ocean of my diet, instructing me to avoid shellfish, raw eggs, and one other thing that I now cannot remember. Then she prescribed a prenatal vitamin and handed me several sample packets of the enormous bright purple pill. She did a quick vaginal exam, apparently the only one I am going to have until I go into labor, and then the whole thing was over.

The appointment took about twenty-five minutes and she never looked at or touched my stomach. There wasn't time or opportunity to discuss the creeping depression I've been feeling, or how concerned I am about my life changing, or my fear that I won't be able to handle it all. I mean, technically there was. She did ask how I was feeling, but we were going along at such a clip, I couldn't imagine what would happen if I bogged things down with my actual thoughts. She did say she had several patients who stayed on antidepressants through their pregnancies with no side effects whatsoever. That was helpful, considering I've been gnashing my teeth to stubs every night worrying about the implications of taking them: Am I going to burn in hell or give my kid epilepsy?

She also said, somewhere in between the questions about my family's health history and the exam, that she's looking forward to delivering my baby. And that she hopes I won't do something silly, like have a home birth.

Uh-huh.

After the prenatal, I indulged in my bimonthly luxury of getting my eyebrows and toes done. Just as I was lying down, Yelena, who has been in charge of my eyebrows for the last three years, asked how old I am and if I am planning to have children. I hesitated just a second too long, trying to figure out how to answer, and she said, You're pregnant! And I said, Yes, and she said, I knew it! And then we both laughed and I told her how nauseated and tired and freaked out I am, and she told me about her clients who come in to the salon the day before their due date to get a Brazilian bikini wax. Apparently, they want to look good for the doctors. By the time I left, my toes were a lovely lilac and I was laughing my head off.

May 6

The mood swings are so intense. I woke up at four in the morning and scribbled this on the back of a paper bag:

I am eight weeks pregnant and terrified. Each
morning I wake up filled with a peculiar blend of dread
and longing. Who am I, and what the hell is happening to
me? Already I eat uncontrollably, craving foods I
classified as off-limits years ago: huge balls of mozzarella,
thick steaks dripping with blood, slice after slice of
eggplant. After only eight weeks, my breasts are painful
to the touch, my small nipples now engorged to
twice their normal size and dark as blackberries. I cannot
drive to the store without having to slow the car to twenty
in a fifty-mile-per-hour zone, without pulling over at a
gas station to let the ocean of nausea subside. To make
matters worse, I can no longer get into my favorite pair of
jeans, and my hard-won good posture, the result of
hundreds of Alexander Technique lessons, seems
frightfully on the sway. And oh yeah, forget about planes,
which I have to board every other week to give lectures,
readings, and writing workshops. Just the words "jet"
and "fuel" send me running for the toilet.
    And that's just my body. Far worse is what my mind is
doing to me. In my worst moments, when I am seeing my
patient and adoring partner as a modern-day Satan, and
feeling as if I am going to be an unfit joke of a mother, I
am certain that I am being invaded by alien intelligence, a

force so powerful it can make me do things I otherwise would not, a force so totally in control of me, I may never know who I am again. And while daddy-to-be can make eggs and burn the turkey bacon just like I like it, he can't really help with the psychological plunges I keep having to claw my way out of because after all, I am going to be this child's mother, and heaven help me and her if I can't figure out how to contain my anxiety about it. Right?

Of course, being the writer and reader and info-junkie that we all are these days, I've bought a half-dozen books to try to get myself through this. I've scoured all 669,801 pages on the Internet on pregnancy and the first trimester, pregnancy and depression, pregnancy and emotions, pregnancy and anxiety, pregnancy and fear. They all, every one of them, allow for the kinds of mood swings I am having, they all say that everything I am feeling and thinking is normal, healthy, and won't hurt the baby. But while the experts say what I want to hear, they still don't seem to say it as adamantly as I need them to. They don't say, Yes, you may feel as if you are going to lose your mind and there will be moments when you reconsider everything and think, after all this wanting and trying and hoping and thinking about names and strollers and birthing methods, that the only reasonable thing to do at this point is terminate the pregnancy.

They don't tell you that. Or if they do, they tell you in tones so soft and modest and reserved and professional that you want to scream at the page, the computer, the doctor, Yes, but do you understand that this whole thing is *freaking me out?* My life is about to change and *I have no idea how to prepare?* And do you know why they are calm and you are not? Because they don't have to have this baby, you do. They are not going to be responsible for this being for the rest of their lives, you are. They are not going to lie in bed worrying about the week of doxycycline you took before you knew you were pregnant and whether or not the baby is going to have stained teeth that need forty thousand dollars' worth of veneers. They are going to go home at the end of the day without carrying your baby with them. You will never be able to go home at the end of the day without carrying your baby again.

Cheery, huh?

May 7

Went to see the Tibetan doctor I have been trying to get an appointment with for months. She's in town for only four or five days every two weeks. Her office was in a cramped suite at the top of a dark stair in a nondescript building on an exceedingly plain street. I chatted a little with a woman in a wheelchair in the waiting room, who told me she has been seeing the doctor for years and swears by her. Everyone else I talk to about her says the same thing. That she comes from a long line of doctors—her father is one of the Dalai Lama's private physicians—and she's incredible.

After forty-five minutes, she appeared and invited me into the inner office. I sat at the foot of the examination table in a wooden chair and told her I was pregnant and super-nauseated and super-tired and maybe just a tiny bit more anxious than usual. She nodded and took my pulse. Then I said, Well, maybe I am way more anxious than usual, and a bit depressed, and she nodded again and asked me to stick out my tongue. She asked me a few more questions about my diet and what times of the day I feel best and worst.

Then she said that there is still a chance I can lose the baby, and that I should keep my stomach and the rest of my body warm. She gave me a list of warming foods to eat, and herbal pellets to quiet the nausea, ease the anxiety, and clear my system of damp, cold, and clogging elements. She told me to make a drink of pomegranate juice, ginger tea, and honey, and to take 300 mg of liquid magnesium a day. She said I should consider going off the antidepressant.

Uh, really?

When I came out carrying my little silk bags of herbs and a sheaf of instructions, Glen was waiting for me. He was skeptical about the herbs. He wanted to make sure they wouldn't hurt the baby. I got upset and told him that this doctor has been treating people for years and years and that I didn't think she would give me something that would damage the baby. I told him what she said about the antidepressant, and he said I should choose one doctor and follow him or her. He said that all of this doctor-hopping was really just a manifestation of my fear of my life changing and how overwhelming and uncontrollable it all is. He said that if I am not careful, I could end up hurting myself or the baby, or both.

I burst into tears.

He may be right, but it's weird to have to listen to someone else's concerns about what I do with my body. Even though I get theoretically that it's Glen's baby, too, at the moment it's still a bit abstract. Yesterday he reminded me, after I called the baby mine one too many times, that I *am* appearing on national TV and radio promoting my latest book on masculinity and saying that men need to be more involved with every aspect of domestic life and women need to let them.

Which made me wonder, am I being a hypocrite when I think, Just let me deal with the baby in my body, you go get food and protect me while I'm doing it? It feels sacrilegious to think it, blasphemous to write it down, but maybe there is something to this whole biology thing.

Needless to say, I had a splitting headache by the time I got home. I took three of my new pellets, one of each kind. I had to crack one of them open with my teeth and chew it up. It tasted like dirt mixed with, I don't know, cyanide?

I HAVE BEEN sleeping for eight hours and now I am *starving*. I find the incessant desire to eat, no matter how shitty I am feeling, both fascinating and annoying. It's as if the baby doesn't care what I am going through, she's going to make it here no matter what.

May 8

On what I can already tell is going to be the first of many out-ings in search of pregnancy clothes that don't make me look like an infantilized suburban housewife, today I went to a shop called Japanese Weekend. It was recommended by one of my more stylish friends, and so it was in anticipation of the Prada of maternity wear that I made my way up Powell Street. What I found was a modest shop with six or seven racks of black, white, denim, and khaki pants and one Asian-styled top in several cheery prints.

At first I was disappointed. I just couldn't get excited about the same plain pants in four colors, all with a thick elastic band around the waist. But then Blanca, the very gentle and attentive saleswoman, suggested I try the pants in a small changing room and nodded approvingly at my reflection when I did. As she admired, I berated myself for being such a snob. The pants were fantastic, and I decided in a matter of seconds that I was never taking them off.

In my determination to "network with other moms to ensure the success of my baby," as advised by the editors of the *Fit Pregnancy* magazine I scoured in my ob/gyn's waiting room, I started talking to the other trying-to-stay-cool mamas trying on pants. One woman was five months "along" and had a gigantic one-year-old knocked out in a stroller. Even though she couldn't stop herself from telling me that her son was in the ninety-fifth percentile for weight and height for his age group, I was terribly impressed with this mom. She was dressed casually, in a simple black T-shirt and jeans, and had her dark, curly hair pulled back in a ponytail. She was confident and friendly and seemed very down to earth. She had great cheekbones and lovely lips that were lightly rouged.

Because she wasn't the total mess I expect a woman with a baby in a stroller and one on the way to be, I asked for her secret.

She said humor and a stay-at-home husband. Then she began extolling the virtues of the Japanese Weekend pant, namely the elastic band that sits below the belly and can be folded over in the later months. I fell more in love with her when she called the pants she was looking for a "piece," and then pulled the pants she thought would be good for me from the sale rack.

The second mom-to-be to share the mirror was a little more high-strung. She looked like a corporate lawyer on her lunch break, and she tore through the options Blanca handed her with alacrity. We asked each other what I have surmised to be the stock mom-to-be questions: How many months, is this your first, do you know if it's a girl or a boy, and have you picked a name? She was four months pregnant with her first, a girl, with no name. When I congratulated her and said, "Oh how exciting, you're having a girl!" she grimaced and said, "Well, I don't know, girls are easier in the beginning but much harder later on. You know, the whole mother-daughter thing." I was so shocked by her candor that I just nodded and ducked back into the dressing cubicle. But I can't stop thinking about what she said. I just want my baby to be healthy, but I know what she means.

May 9

Mother's Day.

Went with my mother to see a documentary about a guy who eats McDonald's food for thirty days. After the film, I told her that I've been feeling depressed, and she told me she was depressed throughout her pregnancy. She said that she always assumed it was because she was isolated in Mississippi, where I was born and where she was working with my father in the civil rights movement, but maybe it was hormonal and genetically so. She said she was practically suicidal, and there were days and days she couldn't get out of bed. She said between the nausea (check) and the depression (double check), she almost lost her mind.

When I spoke with my father on the phone last night, he confirmed her memory. I asked how he dealt with it, and he said, Well, it was hard. Then he told me a story I'd never heard:

My mother wanted to go to Mexico after her first trimester because she was convinced that the sun and getting out of Mississippi would make her feel better. The only problem was that they didn't have any money. So my father put their car, the VW Bug his mother bought him when he graduated from law school, up for sale. *Your car?* I screech. You sold *your car* to go on a trip to Mexico? He laughs, not quite able to believe it, either. We lived in a suburb. My father's office was blocks and blocks away, as was the grocery store and just about everything else. He said it seemed so important to my mother, and he knew he could get a loaner from work. So they sold the Bug and went to Mexico, where they bought two paintings by the now famous Mexican painter Rufino Tamayo and got nauseated riding on public buses careening around mountain curves.

I asked my father if my mother's depression lifted as a result of the trip. I think I remember a picture of her in Mexico, wearing a red-and-white serape and a huge smile. He is silent for a long moment. You know, Rebec, I can't remember. I don't think so.

Shit.

May 12

I broke the bank today at the market. I bought three different kinds of prenatal vitamins, two bottles of nausea-quelling ginger syrup, a box of healthy-pregnancy tea, two whole cooked chickens, two dozen eggs, bunches and bunches of kale, spinach, and broccoli, a huge piece of halibut, two containers of tuna, two Caesar salads, two containers each of blueberries and strawberries, tomatoes, carrots, and about six different kinds of organic chocolate, including a pound of fruit-sweetened chocolate-covered raisins. I have no doubt that if I had more arms, time, and money, I would have filled five more carts. I can't tell if I was hungry, slightly manic, or revved up with pregnancy hormones.

I rushed home to meet Sonam, my potential midwife, whom I have known for years and always imagined delivering my baby. She arrived with her granddaughter asleep in a stroller just as I was unpacking the last grocery bag, took her shoes off, and asked if she could brush her teeth. Then we sat around my kitchen table with a calendar trying to figure out how pregnant I am. I told her Dr. Lowen's estimate of eight weeks from the ultrasound, and that I think I am more like ten weeks. She took notes about how I have been feeling (tired, nauseated, depressed) while I made tea and devoured a container of tuna and a whole box of crackers.

When her granddaughter woke up, we shifted into the bedroom and talked some more while the baby went around the bedroom picking up my shoes and letting them fall to the floor with a boom that made her laugh. It was great to have a real live baby in the house, a prelude to what is to come. Since Sonam is a friend of both my mother and me, and because she asked, I told her that my mom wasn't as enthusiastic as I had hoped. She told me to remember that whatever is going on with my mother has nothing to do with me, and that babies have a way of transforming families. She also said depression is common, especially in the first trimester, and that I should boost my vitamin B intake to help.

Then, get this, I lay down on *my very own* bed, and she felt my stomach, measuring the size of my uterus by counting thumb-widths from my belly button. The second she put her hands on my belly, I knew that I wanted her to deliver the baby. It was like she was talking to the baby with her hands, and the baby was listening. And I felt so safe, like I could fall apart and scream and cry and freak out with her, and she would know what to do.

Lying there, I thought more about how much I want to have this baby at home. The one video of a birth I have seen is of a woman giving birth to her baby in a hot tub with just her husband attending. She goes into labor and she's totally calm, doing deep breathing and walking around their house looking like she's in another dimension. As the contractions get more intense, she hangs on her husband's shoulders and he massages her back. Then she gets into the hot tub and out comes the baby, looking unbothered and serene.

My mother said she wished that my birth could have been like that, instead of in the newly desegregated hospital with the doctor she didn't like, who gave her an episiotomy she may not have needed. My mother's experience haunts me. I am terrified of being cut. Episiotomy, C-section, I just don't want to be lying there helpless and at the mercy of a bunch of doctors in a hurry to get to their golf game.

May 14

I flew to Seattle yesterday to keynote the annual benefit dinner for the Northwest Women's Law Center. I talked about how since I've been pregnant, I've been more concerned than ever about the need for people in politics and the public eye to have healthy personal lives. So often the momentous cultural work happens at the expense of family and sustained intimacy with loved ones. I saw a lot of heads nodding as I spoke, and several couples came up afterward to talk about their experiences trying to keep their families together in the midst of giving so much of themselves to the work they care about.

I met some interesting people at the dinner, including a judge who told me about the evisceration of the Equal Employment Opportunity Commission, and the loveliest woman who was seven months pregnant. Of course we had a pregnancy moment because I can't stop myself from telling every single person I meet my news, and pregnant women? Forget it. It's all I can do not to grab them and sit them down in a corner somewhere to pump them for info about the road ahead. The vast, miraculous wilderness of gestation is my new frontier. I'm looking ahead, gathering provisions. I think I'm becoming a mother.

The woman's name was Anna and this is her second pregnancy; she lost her first child last year to a rare disease. She had sadness in her eyes for the one she lost, but excitement in her laugh for the one to come. I got choked up talking to her. She was inspiring and vulnerable, and I wanted to hug her and take care of her and marvel at her. I was a mess. She lost her child, and then summoned the faith to do it all over again. How do human beings do it?

May 18

Stayed up all night finishing a book review of a new Audre Lorde biography I agreed to write months ago. What a fascinating life. At one point she had a husband, two kids, and a wife—my kind of woman! But she also had major issues: a raging temper, self-absorption that wasn't easy on her kids or lovers. I am determined to live in a way that puts my baby first. I would rather not have a child than subject another human being to eking out an identity in the wake of unbridled narcissism.

But are narcissists aware of their narcissism? I could be going along la-di-da, thinking everything is fine, oblivious to how my choices are impacting my child. I have to rely on Glen to keep me on track. Last night he told me for the umpteenth time that being a parent is easy if you put the needs of the children first. If we can figure out what is best for them and do that, he says, we'll be okay.

May 19

Super-depressed and nauseated today. Can't eat. Keep having sick fantasies that the baby is going to be deformed and Glen is going to have a freak accident and leave me to raise the baby alone. I spent hours looking at the listings the realtor sent over. Two-bedroom unrenovated houses for a million dollars. My deformed child and I are going to live in a shack.

Definitely depression. I'll be puttering away, feeling fine about it all, and then, wham! The undertow.

May 20

Long day. Depressed in the morning, but managed to eke out an hour or so of writing. I forgot the second thing depression takes from me: productivity.

Had lunch with a writer friend in the afternoon. While we were waiting for our udon, Tina told me about her pregnancy: She was twenty-one, alone, and barely out of foster care. She ate M&M's all day and taught herself how to be a parent by reading Dr. Spock. She said she was too proud and too angry to say she needed help and ended up alone and depressed.

I am not sure why, given what she told me, but I asked if she wanted another child. She said absolutely not, no, never. She had preeclampsia, a pelvic cavity not big enough for the baby, and a C-section. She was left with stretch marks all over her body and a baby who at six weeks had to have an operation because he wouldn't stop projectile vomiting.

I got it, but as she was talking I kept thinking about her son, Mark. He is absolutely gorgeous. Smart and athletic. Sweet. The last time I saw him, he was wearing khakis and a white sweater and looked like a movie star. He hugged his mom and kissed her on the cheek. It just doesn't seem possible that he could be the result of such a hideous experience, and yet there it is: the contradiction at the core of the whole endeavor.

A documentary on celibacy was on a few nights ago, and in it, a psychiatrist talked about the urge to procreate and how it is the strongest human urge, stronger even than the urge to eat. That will to multiply—the sheer force of it leaves me speechless. Take this one in my belly. He is determined to be here. I can feel the force of his being. It's as if he has something to do here and just wants to arrive and grow up so he can get to it. *He's* not ambivalent at all.

On the way home, I stopped by my mother's house and shook my head as she dismissed my concerns about money and affordable housing for the baby. *Easy for her to say,* I thought. She's got four huge, beautiful houses. I had to remind her that when she was pregnant with me, my father had already bought their house and was supporting her utterly and completely, an option never presented to me, as a baby feminist, as feasible. Letting a man support me while I nest and think positive thoughts, that is.

Anyway.

Leaving her house, I was compelled to do a little retail therapy. Of course, the whole time I was shopping I was thinking that once the baby comes I will never shop again because I will have to pay for diapers and child care and car seats and bottles and blankets.

The thought was like walking into an airplane propeller.

May 21

Went to see Marie. She agrees with Glen that because of the hereditary predisposition to pregnancy-related depression (and because of the mood swings, three-hour crying spells, and thoughts so horrible I feel ashamed to even write them down), I should consider increasing the dose of my antidepressant. Even though I troll the Internet almost every night looking for articles on the impact of antidepressants on babies, I felt relief just hearing her say the words.

I know that between the two of us, the baby is the most vulnerable right now and I need to do everything I can to protect her, but I have to take care of myself, too. I feel selfish and guilty, but also self-aware and proud. I haven't succumbed to the cultural pressure to sacrifice my hard-won sanity if it isn't absolutely necessary. I'm still a whole human being with needs. I'm an equal partner in this baby equation.

I'm agonizing over untold possibilities, but I feel fortunate to live at a time when depression is recognized as a treatable illness rather than, say, a religious or criminal defect. At least a few people understand that the choice I'm making isn't frivolous, it's necessary.

May 23

Dreamed last night about my ex-boyfriend Andrew, but I think I was really dreaming about all of the guys I have loved but didn't have children with. In the dream, Andrew and I were driving down a narrow road. It was overcast. Huge limestone churches and tiny houses covered with thatch came in and out of focus out the window. I was talking, and kept touching Andrew's hand as he moved the gear stick. He nodded and looked at me at all the right moments, but responded to me in Russian. Guttural, emphatic, lightning-fast Russian. I thought to myself that I must know how to speak his language and I cycled through all of the languages I know bits and pieces of, but could find no Russian. It dawned on me that we had no way to communicate, and that we had been this way for a very, very long time. I didn't flinch, and calmly kept stroking Andrew's hand, but I thought to myself that our relationship was over, and that everything was about to change.

This must have something to do with the e-mail I got from Andrew a few days ago. I have been thinking so much about our five-year relationship and what went wrong. The last time I saw him, he was living in Japan and teaching English. I traveled twenty hours to visit him, and after four days of wandering through temples in Kyoto and two days on a ferry to Shikoku, we had a huge, melodramatic fight complete with screaming and slamming doors and walking out of apartments in the middle of the night.

I ended up fleeing back to Narita airport in Tokyo in a taxi that cost three hundred dollars, driven by an officious man wearing white gloves and a little black cap. I didn't understand a word he said, but every ten minutes he would catch my eye in the rearview mirror and say, Narita? And I would look back at him and say, Yes, Narita. And he would say, Okay.

I can't remember what Andrew and I fought about, but I have missed knowing, over these last ten years, whether he is alive or dead, happy or miserable. Within forty-eight hours of Googling him, I was staring at photos of his beautiful wife and daughter. They are living in Hawaii; Andrew is weeks away from his Ph.D. In his note he sounded the same. Same dry British-American wit, same Sephardic warmth. I told him about the baby and he congratulated me. He said he always knew I would be a wonderful mother.

I woke up this morning feeling the distance between my life now and all the people I still love but no longer know. After a lifetime filled with a seemingly endless array of choices, I'm somewhat stunned to find myself making such a definitive one. It's thrilling to be opening the door to a new life with Glen, but terrifying to be shutting all the other doors to all the other lives. A part of me wants to leave an escape route open, some ember from an old flame smoldering, just in case. But another part says, No, this is it, you have a child to think about now, and turns away.

Three

LIKE MANY WOMEN MY AGE, I spent a good deal of time and energy trying not to have a baby. I may be speaking too broadly here, but I don't think so. Mine is the first generation of women to grow up thinking of children as optional, a project that might pan out to be one of many worthwhile experiences in life, but also might not. We learned that children were not to be pursued at the expense of anything else. A graduate degree in economics, for example, or a life of renunciation, devoted to a Hindu mystic. To live life as one long series of adventures in "sexual freedom" could be added to the list, along with becoming president, or at least secretary of state.

I don't remember exactly how these ideas were transmitted, but that I imbibed them is unquestionable. It must have had something to do with my mother being a cultural icon, and the private carryover of her public insistence that even one child

could, if not managed properly, erode one's hard-won independence. In an oft-quoted essay she wrote as a young mother, she
remembers her mother's admonition to have a second child as
uncharacteristically bad advice. In a poem written around the
same time, she compares me to various calamities that struck and
impeded the lives of other women writers. Virginia Woolf was
mentally ill and the Brontës died prematurely. My mother has
me, whom she lists as a delightful distraction, but by context and
comparison, it's clear I was a calamity just the same.

The effect of living with my mother's ambivalence about the
role of children in a woman's life, the role of *me* in her life, could
not bode well for me having my own. Ambivalence itself is rarely
positive. Ambivalence about one's offspring is a horrific kind of
torture for all involved. It affects me to this day, stealing my certi-
tude at critical moments. I have sat with others and said, Well, of
course my mother loves me. But in the very next moment I will
purse my lips and squint my eyes and tilt my head back and
remember all of the indices of ambivalence, and the thought will
arise with an even greater clarity: or maybe she does not.

People who cannot conceive of parental ambivalence have a
very difficult time understanding this, and write it off as the confusion and ingratitude of children. But this is the price of ambivalence over a lifetime: It doesn't go away. It seeps into otherwise
healthy tissue and tinges it with seeds of pathology. Does my
mother love me unconditionally? Will it be possible to love my
own child this way?

There was also the veiled competition that throbbed between
my mother, an extremely driven artist determined to be successful on her own terms in a decidedly antagonistic world, and my

stepmother, an equally educated woman who, more than anything else, wanted to give birth to and raise five children. I can't
say that these two did not get along, because in order for this to
be true they would have had to spend time with each other, and
they only met four times in thirty years. But their respective
choices, the extremely divergent ways they constructed and displayed their femininity, loomed large in my mind. So large that
the tension between the two of them as individuals, typical
stepmother–birth mother tensions, with the added challenges of
being from different races and socioeconomic backgrounds, was
transformed in my psyche as a tension between ways of being a
woman.

Because these things are impressed upon us often before we
realize we have a mind that can be impressed upon, I instinc-
tively felt that I must be loyal to my mother's version. This meant
maintaining my autonomy at all costs. To stop working and raise
children, to be weighed down with tots like so many anvils
around my neck, none of these were acceptable. They smelled of
betrayal and a lack of appreciation for the progress made on
behalf of women's liberation. Worse, they suggested a kind of
ignorance about the truth of the gendered world, which was that
unless women refuse, their children would enslave them. Which
was that the myth of blissful motherhood was just that, a myth,
and the reality was much more banal.

The only problem with this program was my stepmother. She
wasn't especially well known or respected in her field, and she
too, as a stepmother, had her share of ambivalence about being in
a relationship with me. But my stepmother brought maternal
enthusiasm and predictability to my life. She was enthusiastic

about children in general and being a parent specifically, and predictable in that I could count on her to be the neurotic and intrusive maternal figure that Jewish mothers are often characterized as being. While my own mother could be counted on to recommend a life-changing book and to take me to a fascinating but remote village in Indonesia, my stepmother could be counted on to keep the refrigerator stocked with low-fat but tasty food, and to bring at least one camera to all events at which any of her children were to be featured.

Because divorce was not yet the exhausted psychological terrain it is today, there were no adults in my life who had the wherewithal to identify my dilemma and help me navigate it. There was no one who said to me, the way we now say to kids who are mixed race or bi-religious or have two daddies, Isn't it wonderful that you have these two role models and they are both so different! No one said over and over again (because that's how many times it takes) or even once, When you grow up you can embrace motherhood wholeheartedly and still accomplish great things. It seems absurdly obvious now, but growing up, I swear, I could not fathom it.

I dealt with the impossibility of my predicament by pretending it didn't exist. I made the requisite strides toward personal fulfillment through professional achievement, telling myself that I would think about having a baby when the time was right. Because I believed that there would be several if not dozens of other possible partners, at twenty I abandoned the first man with whom I could actually imagine having children, and didn't make another serious attempt until ten years later.

At the time I abandoned him, I felt relieved. Then I felt sad and despondent. Then I began to dream that my breasts were being chopped off with a huge machete. Constantly. Every day. By the time I got to therapy, I had seen my breasts chopped off at least ten thousand times. By the time I realized, also in therapy, that it was my own hand on the knife, I was already deep into another relationship, infusing it with the same ambivalence. Did I want a husband, children? Did I want to be free and empowered to do whatever I wanted? Was the latter just a ruse to sabotage the former?

The ambivalence reared its head, this time with a slightly different presentation. I began to tell people hesitantly, Yes, I do want kids, but I am afraid. Afraid? the person or persons would reply. Of what? Hurting them, I would say. And then they might look at me with surprise or shock or understanding, and I would feel a twinge of shame and sadness, and then we would go on talking about something else, as if nothing was wrong or odd or out of the ordinary whatsoever.

Although it may have been risky, I wish someone had told me right away and with great emphasis, It is okay to worry, but don't by any means let it keep you from having a child! Instead of telling me that I had plenty of time, or that I should adopt because the world is full of needy children, someone should have sat me down, looked me right in the eye, and told me not to let anything keep me from the experience. Trust me, they could have said, barring disease, famine, and the potential for life-threatening violence or financial ruin, no matter what your trepidation, just do it.

They could have shared some version of what my gynecologist told me fifteen years later: "I've delivered thousands of babies, and as a rule, women don't regret having children, they regret not having them."

It is shocking to think that not one person suggested that my fear of hurting my children might really have been a fear of growing up and following my own (not my mother's) belief system.

Because the fact is that until you become a mother, you're a daughter. The fact is that when you almost die so that someone else can live, you become a much larger human being. The fact is that none of the ideas we've gleaned about motherhood from the mothers we know and the mothers we watch on TV mean anything at all because motherhood is in the doing, not the thinking about. Motherhood is brand-new every time; motherhood is full of possibility. Just like when John and Yoko said "War Is Over." Motherhood Is Free.

If you want it.

May 24

Spoke with my artist friend Sarah today. She gets the prize for the most foot-in-mouth response: You're pregnant? Oh my God, congratulations! My friend just had a miscarriage.

After an awkward pause, I said, Yeah, well, I'm not going to be having one of those, thank you very much, and then we both cracked up.

I've been getting e-mails from all over and they are all so beautiful and supportive. Yesterday Rikke wrote that I shouldn't worry, there is a reason it takes nine months to give birth: That's how long it takes for the reality of it to set in.

May 26

We got to Mendocino last night to find that a mouse has eaten through all of my clothes. I came up to bed and found one arm of my black sweater, chewed off as perfectly as a piece cut from a dress pattern, lying on the floor. We've got to get a cat. Or call Terminix.

On the way up from the city, Glen and I got into a huge argument about the birth and who will attend. My fantasy is that everyone I know and love will climb into the hot tub-cum-birthing pool with me. They will rub my legs and massage lavender essential oil into my scalp. Those who don't want to be in the water, or need a break from the festivities, will take shifts operating the iPod, or cooking. Every half hour I will be offered a fresh serving of pasta with garlic and oil, or organic chocolate cake. When the baby is born, everyone will say a blessing from a different spiritual tradition before we cut the cord.

Glen thinks my polytheistic fiesta theme is unrealistic and unsafe and doesn't honor the primacy of our relationship. He said he refused to be a part of a birth that was more than five miles from a hospital. He kept asking where we, as a couple, fit into my vision. Is there anything that is only for us? he wanted to know. Had I considered the impact that sharing such a major event will have on our intimacy as a couple? And what if something goes wrong? Do we really want that many people in the middle of such a critical moment?

He made some good points, but I wasn't ready to hear them. Instead I launched into a tirade about how it is *my* birth experience, and it should be however *I* want it to be, and how *dare* he even ask about *us*. For God's sake, I yelled, we have the rest of our lives to be together, why on earth should we be so *precious* and *controlling* about the birth? And anyway, I yelled, *studies show* that women surrounded by family and friends have shorter, *easier* labors. To which Glen replied, Well, that's great, but have there been any *studies* on the *divorce rates* for those women?

After a few minutes of strained silence, I had a flash of the baby and how arguments like these might frighten him or her, if they don't already. I thought about something Glen and I have talked a lot about: not arguing, and prioritizing peace between us over whatever ideas our intellects have gotten hooked on. I never want ideology or "being right" to take precedence over loving one another and being a family. There's just too much to lose. The baby's mental health and Glen himself are just a couple of things that come to mind.

And so I am rethinking the birth plan, and telling the little voice that wants everything her way that she has to be open. You're not alone anymore, I keep telling her. And that's a good thing. Yeah, right, she says, and turns her face the other way.

Before we went to bed, we talked about names. I've been calling the baby Milarepa, after a Buddhist ascetic who tamed both human beings and animals by singing to them.

Maybe we should name the cat Milarepa. Or the mouse.

May 28

Carl came over to look at the water heater this morning. Turns out it is "pretty ancient," and mineral deposits have built up inside the tank, taking up all the room where the hot water should go. He said it's a fire hazard, and that by the way, when he was looking at the heater he noticed that the main supporting beams under the bathhouse also need replacing. This last alert evoked a gruesome image of the building collapsing and pitching the baby and me out of the bathtub and into a patch of poison ivy.

After he left, I did two phone interviews from last week that Leslie, my publicist, rescheduled for today. The first interviewer was a young woman from Detroit who "loved" the latest collection of essays I've edited, *What Makes a Man: 22 Writers Imagine the Future.* She asked questions about the contributors, the importance of looking critically at masculinity, and the relationship between this book and *To Be Real: Telling the Truth and Changing the Face of Feminism,* an anthology about Third Wave feminism I edited ten years ago.

The second interviewer was an ex-Marine who claimed that male aggression is biological, that men who don't believe this are gay, and that I am offending our armed forces by questioning male aggression while our country is at war. When I told him that we probably had more in common than he thought, he said that no, he didn't think so. I said, Well, I am going to bet that we both want peace, and that neither of us wants our children to be killed in war. He said that war is necessary for democracy, and that he would be willing to sacrifice his child for the preservation of the American way of life.

Who knows? He might be right about all of it, but when he said he'd be willing to sacrifice his child, a huge wave of exhaustion came over me. I felt that if I didn't lie down that very second, I might collapse. I exited as politely as I could, made for the kitchen, and scarfed the entire pot of soup Glen made last night. Then I climbed up the little ladder to bed and fell asleep.

It's now four in the morning. I have been sleeping for almost ten hours, but I still have the voice of the interviewer in my head. For what would I be willing to sacrifice my child?

June 1

Arrived at JFK in New York for the first time with baby on board. Everything was different because now all I can see are the women with babies. Were they always there? I am obsessed with how they move. Are they alone or do they have help? What kind of stroller are they pushing? Do they have a purse *and* a diaper bag? Cute or sensible shoes? Do cabdrivers do anything special to make it easier for them? Do they look happier than the childless women teetering by in high-heeled Manolos?

Now at my father's house on the Upper East Side, getting ready for the long drive tomorrow to see Solomon, the now fourteen-year-old young man I've been helping to raise since he was eight, at boarding school. Since his mother and I broke up, we've been trading off visiting days. I get the two days before his graduation from ninth grade, she gets actual graduation and the day after.

In what seems to be yet another manifestation of my ambivalence affliction, I can't figure out if I should tell Sol about the baby. I remember how abandoned I felt when my stepmother told me she was going to have her own biological child. The least I can do is spare him those feelings during a time that's supposed to be all about him and his accomplishments. On the other hand, I am pretty sure I'm showing, and I don't want him to figure it out and have to ask.

Pondering this, I feel an awful conflagration of elation and dread. I think I already love this little being inside of me more than I've ever loved anyone. How will this affect this person I consider to be, in many ways, my first child, the son I didn't give birth to but whom I adore nonetheless?

June 2

Arrived in Lake Placid after a long drive out of the city. I hung out with Solomon at his school for the evening, eating and talking to his housemates and a few other parents who came up early for graduation. I heard about miles hiked, potatoes harvested, accidents sustained while snowboarding, and "hook-ups." I was regaled with a *very* graphic description of the three a.m. birth of a lamb, and told that I am one of the coolest parents because I am young and wear "cool" clothes.

I like these kids. Over the last couple of years, I've watched them give presentations in their biology and Spanish classes, and even take stabs at improv. I've talked to their parents and grandparents, and heard their personal stories, many of them difficult. I am always in awe of how happy they seem in this environment. How the intimate, back-to-the-land, child-centered learning philosophy brings out their shiny, forceful natures.

Now that I am pregnant, I can't help but wonder if this place had something to do with it. There's a utopic feeling here, kids and adults together in the wilderness, planting, harvesting, learning, playing. I've liked knowing Sol is here, safe through the trials of 9/11 and largely unaware of its aftermath. Driving back to the hotel, I thought, Well, if I sink into a depression that threatens to damage my child, or if I buckle under the pressure of balancing the demands of work with the constant labor of motherhood, or if Glen leaves me and never wants to see me or his child again and I'm devastated, there's always boarding school. It sounds awful, but the thought was infinitely reassuring.

I told Sol about the baby within the first hour, after I caught him checking out my waistline. He was excited and immediately told his favorite houseparent, who, in addition to being a total Macintosh devotee, is a caring, gentle guy. I took his excitement as a sign that I haven't wrecked his graduation moment, and that the whole biological, nonbiological sibling thing just might work out.

June 3

I drove over to the school and spent the whole day. I asked Sol to take me to his favorite places on campus, the places he will miss the most. He took me on a trail through the woods to an old tree house, and then I followed him to the other side of the campus, to the tents around the lake. We stood there for a few minutes, getting lost in the shimmering water and wide-open sky.

Solomon will stay with me tonight at the hotel, and in the morning I will take him back to school and say goodbye. I am sad I will miss his departure speech, but I believe this way is best for everyone. In addition to the other complex dynamics of the day, including the presence of Solomon's biological father whom I don't really know, I feel protective of the baby. I don't want him or her to, for one second, get caught up in the emotional aftermath of the separation from Solomon's mother I've worked so hard to put behind me.

When I asked Solomon how he felt about the split schedule, he gave me his usual "Why are you always asking me how I *feel*?" look, and said it was fine.

I'm afraid it's the best I can do and, for once, I can live with that.

June 4

I love New York: the movement, the fashion, the dynamism. The heady mix of high and low. It's like a drug. Whenever I visit, I have to brace myself for the wave of ambivalence about California that washes over me. I miss the endless IV drip of films, performances, plays, and shopping. Food delivery of any kind at any time. Tasti D-Lite. Fortunately, I've been on this roller coaster enough times to know that in another forty-eight hours I'll start getting tired and missing the more reasonable rate of stimulation of the other coast. In seventy-two hours I will be pining for home.

I am happy to report that it's a little easier to feel good about my decision now that I've got the tot to think about. I want the baby to know New York so intimately that it loses its power to frighten and overwhelm. So intimately that she can harness the power of it for her own dreams. I owe her that. But fighting it out with a stroller on the subway? I just don't see it.

June 5

I have decided to stop using "her" and "she." Yes, I want to counter all of those years of the masculine pronoun standing in for all of humanity, but I really, really know in my heart that I am having a boy. It's the most obvious thing in the world to me. I refuse to allow my political beliefs to trump my intuition because that was the point of all of those political beliefs, wasn't it? To be able to trust our intuition?

June 6

My sister and stepmother took me shopping today for more maternity clothes. My sister took on the role of personal shopper, perusing the racks, and my stepmother was the voice of reason.

It was like being back in junior high, in a good way, until we split up and I tried to brave "the biggest maternity department in the city" by myself. All I got there was a big headache and another crashing wave of depression. Was it the J.Lo blaring through the store's speakers, the haggard-looking mothers being dragged around by whiny, unruly kids, or the upbeat, colorful display of tees I couldn't fit into juxtaposed against maternity wear that looked like it belonged on Dora the Explorer? Hmmm, let me think.

I got so freaked out walking around the store, I had to call Glen just to get my bearings. I know he must have thought I was losing it because I kept saying, Is this what's going to happen to me? Am I going to be trapped behind a stroller for the rest of my life, at the beck and call of some badly behaved toddler screaming for his sippy cup? And will I be wearing beige chinos and an oversized T-shirt with a company logo on it? And will I look and be so tired that I won't even care?

It reminded me of the *Sex and the City* episode when Miranda volunteers to frost her ex-boyfriend's new girlfriend's birthday cupcakes, and she calls Carrie in tears. Carrie's like, Why are you doing that? and Miranda kind of flops around, not knowing what to say. Then Carrie gets serious and tells Miranda to step away from the cupcakes.

After trying to talk me down three or four different ways, Glen finally told me to get out of the store. And even though he was three thousand miles away, and just a bunch of little sound waves coming through a piece of plastic, I did.

June 7

Spent a few hours today having my portrait taken by Marion Ettlinger, who has taken so many amazing author photos. She took the image of Lucy Grealy I like so much, with the bird on her shoulder, and the stunning portrait of Jhumpa Lahiri. Marion was great, warm but not overly so. We talked, but her eyes did most of the work, quietly taking me in. Her studio felt like a writer's study in Paris circa 1920, very Anaïs Nin and Henry Miller, all dark velvet chaises and antique wooden side tables, thirty-five-millimeter cameras and natural light.

While she was shooting, we talked about getting married. She loves her guy and wants to tie the knot, but feels she'd be selling out her feminist roots. I laughed and said, It's official, female ambivalence has reached an all-time high, it's an epidemic! I told her about how long I've wanted a baby and how scared I am. I told her that the only way I've been able to do it has been to choose my persistent, irrational, very human yearnings for close-ness with other human beings over admittedly valuable feminist ideology that wasn't born of my own experience. I asked, If the relationship is healthy, is there ever a reason to let ideology keep us from committing more deeply to the people we love?

I can't say I have the answer, but I do think it's a legitimate question.

When we were done, I headed downtown to my friend Trajal's dance performance. Afterward, a bunch of us went to dinner, where the baby and his name were the main topics of conversa-tion. The response to "Milarepa" was lukewarm, but people liked "Tenzin," after the Dalai Lama, which I've been throwing around for the last few weeks.

Tenzin Walker, our playwright friend Brooke said, that's strong. Trajal took to it right away, and started to include Tenzin in all our future plans. Well, when Tenzin is born, we'll have to have a party, and, I can't wait to go to Paris with Tenzin.

Paris with Tenzin!

I felt like the belle of the ball. Even though it was Trajal's night, being pregnant makes every night my night. Not long ago I heard Dr. Christiane Northrup speaking about yin wisdom, and how the egg waiting for the sperm is full of it. The egg just calls out to the sperm and then waits, knowing the whole school is going to come calling. I feel like that. For the first time in my life, being is effortless. My job is to sit and glow. All I have to do is wait and the whole world, the whole big life experience, is going to come and land right at my feet.

Tenzin Walker!

June 8

Met with John Vaughn today for lunch. He's directing a project for the Twenty-First Century Foundation called the Black Men and Boys Initiative, focusing on the status of African-American men in our culture and what can be done to change it. The statistics are disheartening. Forty percent of African-American men drop out of high school. One in every four is incarcerated. I can't help but think of the assassinations of Martin Luther King, Jr., Medgar Evers, and Malcolm X. The dissolution of the Panthers through COINTELPRO. The marginalization of African-American men in every segment of American culture but hip-hop, jazz, and sports. How few African-American men I see at universities where I speak, supermarkets where I shop, restaurants where I eat. How rarely I see an African-American man on a plane.

Because they are so rare, I know most of the African-American men succeeding in corporate America. Richard Parsons at Time Warner, Kenneth Chenault at American Express. Russell Simmons, important because he has managed to make his millions without wearing a suit and tie, without forfeiting ownership, and without becoming unrecognizable to the people he grew up with, or to himself.

It is as if, in response to the leadership African-American men have displayed, they have been targeted for annihilation, or at least total subordination. It is as if, in response, African-American men have chosen to keep their intellects undercover, or not to develop them at all. Flipping through channels late at night and searching the shelves at the bookstore, I can't believe the glaring absence of African-American intellectualism. But being a brilliant black man can be dangerous, can put you in the crosshairs.

There are the academic superstars: Cornel West and Henry Louis Gates. Michael Eric Dyson. Across the Atlantic, Paul Gilroy. But where is the W.E.B. DuBois, the Frederick Douglass, the Dr. King of our time? The Bayard Rustin and James Baldwin? What happened to credible voices having the power to elucidate, to inspire and inform masses of people? How is it possible that so much of this work of social uplift is left to rap artists who have just barely escaped gangsterism? How is it possible that the African-American intelligentsia seems to have evaporated into the corporate media conglomerate, rarely if ever to be seen or heard providing cogent commentary on the state of affairs? Where are the translators, the people who deconstruct the news to the populace?

Listening to John, I got the feeling they are all in jail. And then I thought, *If I have a boy, how on earth will I protect him?*

June 9

Went to a screening of Spike Lee's film about a man who impregnates lesbians to make ends meet after being fired from a lucrative biotech job. I have to give it to Spike: He takes risks. The film was a little messy, but I don't think people appreciate how far Spike took the discussion within a conservative mainstream context that doesn't want to look at the possible obsolescence of the adult male. Reduced to sperm donors for rich, sexy lesbians? Come on, how easy could that have been to get funded?

I especially liked the scenes in which our hero feels objectified, used, and demoralized during and after sex, a trope usually reserved for women on-screen. It takes a lot of courage to reveal that men have these same anxieties. As they lose a sense of power and control at work and in their personal relationships, their psyches struggle to make the adjustment. I also found myself identifying with the women's intense quest for motherhood, and I appreciated how our hero ultimately partners with two of the women he has impregnated.

It was good to see people I haven't seen in years. Everyone patted my growing belly and seemed genuinely excited for me. Of course I had to pee like a million times and was sweating like I had my own personal sprinkler system hidden beneath my clothes. Have I documented that new side effect? That I get these raging hormonal surges that make me hot and flushed, and dripping with perspiration? It's quite attractive.

Went out to dinner with friends afterward, and then walked sixty blocks back to the apartment. I must be feeling better because my energy is way up and my brain seems to be clear and firing for the first time in weeks. Maybe, just maybe, I am coming out of this damn first trimester into what is supposed to be the fun part. I feel calmer, back to myself, not quite so hysterical and on edge.

Or maybe it's just New York. And the extra dose of the antidepressant Marie prescribed back in San Francisco.

Either way, I talked to Glen as I walked, my boots clicking against the filthy New York pavement, smiling and imagining walking the same city streets with him and the baby.

June 14

Heartbeat! Oh my God. The most outrageous thing I have ever heard. I went in for my second prenatal with Dr. Lowen and, as usual, it was in and out, but the "in" included hearing my baby's heartbeat. Dr. Lowen was completely unimpressed, and she's allowed, considering she hears a gajillion baby heartbeats a day. But I was completely, totally, stupendously overwhelmed. I was floating all over the office. It was all I could do to keep myself from grabbing the Doppler ultrasound and holding it to my stomach for hours.

I am happy to report that the heartbeat is absolutely perfect. Strong, fast, well paced. I took this as another sign that I really do have a baby inside of me. This isn't some vast conspiracy to trick me into believing something that isn't true. In six more months, a real live baby is going to come out of my body and make me a mother. I know, I know, it sounds crazy. But it's true.

To add to my growing distaste for the whole doctor vibe, on my way out the receptionist handed me my "complimentary" diaper bag. It was full of formula samples and coupons for several other baby products. I could take the appreciative and noncynical tack, but I can't believe doctors allow themselves to be the middle-men and -women for these companies. In the intimacy of my doctor's office, where I am, by design, vulnerable and open to her suggestion, seeking it even, I am being marketed to. Am I being too sensitive? It's like commercials at the movies times a hundred.

When I gave the bag back to the nurse, declining politely, she looked at me like I was crazy. Just keep it, she said, you might need it. I just put it on the counter. I don't think so, but thank you so much. Then I worried for an hour that I had come across as an arrogant, ungrateful bitch.

Glen continues to think I should find another OB. He was over Dr. Lowen when we went in for the fertility consultation and she made a remark about men getting bent out of shape when women, "who do so much," ask them to "do a little thing like take a motility test." He felt the remark was insulting, considering all he does, and insensitive, considering the societal mandate that "real men" be virile in the same way that "real women" should be fertile. Even though it isn't a big issue for him, he thinks it is callous for a doctor to miss the fact that motility can be a sore spot for men.

He's right, of course. He totally clocked one of those gynic moments that make me cringe. Moments in which women intent upon "claiming their power" do or say things that belittle the men they say they love.

I mostly agree with Glen about finding another doctor, but the idea of starting the search makes me want to go take a nap. I have been seeing Dr. Lowen for a few years and, I tell Glen with a grin, she's got biracial kids. Glen has accused me of being a sucker for the parents of mixed-race kids more than once. I project noble qualities onto them and make excuses for their bad behavior.

Glen shakes his head. He's not happy that the criteria for staying with the gynecologist who might deliver our baby is her biracial children, but he doesn't revisit the highly contentious discussion we've been having lately about how all of the big baby decisions seem to be made exclusively by me, and I couldn't be more grateful for the respite.

June 22

Had a long discussion with my lobbyist friend Rachel about how many women rely on the samples given to them by their obstetricians because, unlike most developed nations, America has no social support system to speak of for new parents. Paid parental leave, which can be up to two years in countries like Sweden and Denmark and divided between two parents, is virtually nonexistent here, with American women getting only six weeks, if they're lucky. High-quality public child care for preschool-aged children is also the norm in countries like France, but completely unavailable in the United States. New parents have to work long hours to even have a shot at affording excellent child care.

It's hard to understand why our country, one of the wealthiest in the world, seems to care so little about its children. Even from a purely capitalist point of view, you would think that well-looked-after, well-educated children would ensure a competent workforce and stable populace. And studies show that women are able to be more productive with this kind of support, so it's not like we'd lose half the GDP. Rachel thinks it has to do with the low expectations of families in America. Women have been getting six weeks to three months for so long it seems normal, an unquestionable standard.

But I think it also has to do with our cultural ambivalence about the role of biology in women's lives, and how it has been used to suppress and control women. For generations, women have been portrayed as the weaker sex, more emotional and less physically capable than men, and so biologically unsuited for positions of power. In response, women have said no, we aren't biologically anything at all. Shaped more by culture than anatomy, we can be anything we want to be. Tactically, this was a smart move. If women are inherently the same as men, we deserve equal treatment under the law.

Women gained a lot of access using this strategy, but on some fronts, it may have backfired. Case in point: If men and women are inherently equal, and men don't get "special treatment" like extended paternity leave and on-site childcare, why should women? A question that leaves most infants in the arms of hired caregivers instead of their mothers. This strategy has also left women somewhat ambivalent about maternal desire. Is it a biological yearning that should be denied in the name of sameness and women's empowerment? The whole polemic puts women in the ridiculous position of wondering whether wanting a baby is proof that women actually *are* the weaker sex.

I think that parental, rather than maternity, leave is a good way of negotiating this point in the public sphere. We avoid the potentially divisive and ultimately unknowable question of whether women are fundamentally different from men by saying that both parents need and deserve to take care of their children.

But what if we are fundamentally different? Before I got pregnant I would have vehemently rejected this idea. Now I'm not so sure. Now I might try a different tactical approach: Do men and women have to be the same to be treated equally?

I left Rachel's house thinking about what it really means to cut taxes in this country. It means that the bond between parents and children is not supported with programs like extended parental leave, and children's psychosocial and intellectual development is neglected in the absence of decent child care. It also means that many people can't afford to have children at all, let alone provide them with what they need to succeed.

In a country, a world, as rich as ours, this is unacceptable. Reflecting on what this process has meant to me already, in terms of experiencing what it means to be human, I can't help but feel that having children should be a right, not a privilege.

June 23

I met with my midwife Sonam again today. She tested my urine by having me pee on a stick that changed colors, took my temperature, measured my uterus, and listened to the baby's heartbeat with the Doppler, talking to me about baby stuff the whole time. She suggested I start doing prenatal yoga, gave me the names of a couple of teachers she likes, and told me to eat wild salmon and leafy greens. I told her that all I want to do is wander from room to room, have sex, eat, and sleep, and she laughed. That's okay, she said, but remember, labor is a marathon: You have to train. Shoot. You mean I can't just lounge around my boudoir for nine months?

We talked a little business, like what I think about the hospital where she has privileges being public and twenty to thirty minutes away. When I asked what she meant, exactly, by the public part, she said that the hospital is well equipped and has a great neonatal intensive care unit, but serves a very different population than the hospital I usually go to.

She said it's not one-thousand-percent spotless, either. It's an older building and hasn't been renovated. For the most part, the nurses are excellent and she loves her supervising doctor, but the best thing about the place is that she has full privileges there, which means she would be in charge of the birth unless something goes wrong.

What can I say? I wish the public and private hospitals weren't so different. I wish I didn't have to negotiate race and class just to have my baby. I'm going to visit and see how it feels, but I'm pretty sure I'd rather have Sonam deliver this baby in a lean-to than risk having an unnecessary C-section in some spotless shrine to the medical establishment.

At least I think I would.

June 28

Today I met June for lunch. We talked about our new creations: hers, a new publishing venture; mine, the little one growing in my belly. She told me she long ago decided not to have children. She said that several of her friends had children because they thought they should, only to realize too late that they didn't make the decision consciously. Where are they with it now? I wanted to know. They've got kids they don't want, she said, shaking her head.

Yikes.

When I asked more about her decision, she said she didn't feel emotionally able to take care of herself, let alone a defenseless child. Her body was too weak, having weathered a few major illnesses, and her energy too elusive. Her husband wanted kids, but when she asked if it was him or the culture that wanted them he conceded it was the culture. Then she brought her sister's kids home to prove her point. The kids exhausted both her and her husband.

I tried not to get judgmental about her choice. I tried to minimize the whole baby thing and just talk about work stuff, creative stuff, and the machinations of the publishing world. I tried not to gush about how long I have wanted a baby, and how miraculous it is to have another human being growing inside of me.

But it was damn near impossible.

Am I turning into a baby supremacist? One of those people who thinks a woman without a baby is like a fish without an ocean? Who thinks a woman without a baby may be stuck developmentally just shy of true adulthood forever? As June talked about her new office and staff, I thought about how much she's missing and how appalling it is that I can't tell her because the whole thing is so unbelievably primal and indescribable. I thought about how hooked human beings can get on external accomplishment, but how at the moment, the most dramatic and exciting changes of my life are happening inside and I have no desire to go back.

I know I'm setting myself up for some serious refutation, and it's all valid. My thoughts aren't rational. They're hormonal, irrational, psychopharmacological.

And so incredibly real.

Four

IT'S NOT THE SAME. No matter how close you are to your brilliant stepson or beloved stepdaughter, the love you have for your nonbiological child isn't the same as the love you have for your own flesh and blood.

It's different.

I met Solomon when he was seven and I was twenty-six. It was a sunny Los Angeles afternoon, and his mom, whom I had been dating for several weeks, was taking us to the beach. Solomon was wearing blue pants and carried three small action figures. He was quiet and cautious, with intermittent bursts of chattiness. His parents were in the middle of a nasty divorce, and he reminded me of myself at his age, trying to figure out who to be after my parents sat me down and told me their marriage was over.

Within hours of meeting Solomon, I had projected a lifetime

of alienation onto him, ascribing to him all the pain and confusion I felt after my parents ended their marriage. Within weeks I had fallen for him. I loved the way he took my hand when we were out in the city. The way he asked deep and seemingly bizarre questions like, When people die, do they remember who they've been? I loved that he thought he remembered being in his mother's womb and described it as warm, red, and mushy.

Before I even remotely knew whether a relationship with his mother was something I wanted, I dove into Solomon's life and began trying to create the positive post-divorce family I never had. Without thinking it through. Because I thought he needed me. Because I knew my inner seven-year-old needed me. And I had to save her. By saving him.

And so it began. The trips to the orthodontist and ophthalmologist, the monthly talks about schoolwork and conduct with the teachers of third, fourth, fifth, sixth, seventh, eighth, and then, finally, ninth grades. We had the obligatory struggles over homework, diet, and violent video games. I suffered the endless negotiation of the politics, socioeconomic and otherwise, of play dates. I hired helpers, bought and read books on teen sexuality, coalesced and counseled members of the extended family.

I did so much that friends wondered if I wasn't doing too much. I wasn't his *actual* mother, after all. And wasn't it true that if I did too much, I would enable her to do too little? What would happen if his mother and I should break up? Shouldn't I legally adopt him to protect my investment in our relationship? I understood their concerns, but my inner seven-year-old was undaunted. She wanted—no, *needed*—me to keep going.

I wasn't just reparenting myself, though. I was securing my

position in the relationship. Love me, love my kid. That's what single parents say to potential lovers, partners, and spouses. Even when they don't utter the words, it's a running subtext. And don't we potential stepparents respond, if we believe we can make a genuine go of it, with our own subtext? We make dinner for three and watch *Princess Mononoke*. To the exciting new adult in our life we say: Your child is my child. To the adorable child before us we say: I think of you as my own. When we are in deep, and can see that the well-being of another human being is at stake and his ability to trust us *actually matters,* we look straight into his eyes and say: No matter what, I will never leave you.

At least that's what I said. It didn't occur to me that some people would predict a messy endgame and keep their distance. These people would have gone down the "Your child is my child" road with other lovers and friends, only to devastate some unsuspecting kid and get wiped out in the process. But I hadn't yet lost a child, and so I said all of the things I said because I meant them, and because I did not see a way to proceed in the relationship without meaning them. I said them because I had no idea what I was getting myself into. I said them because I was in love and didn't yet know how to think with any organ other than the one in my chest.

In the end I couldn't do it. I couldn't save me and I couldn't save him and I couldn't save her and I couldn't save us. It was an untenable situation and none of us had the skills to make it otherwise. The only thing I can say on our behalf is that we were in our twenties and early thirties and the relationship epitomized our developmental limitations. It was passionate and histrionic, fun and tragic, romantic and stupid.

Being young and coming from families that didn't stay together, we thought if we just loved long and hard enough we could destroy everything a thousand times and put it back together a thousand times, and then one day everything would fall into place. We thought it was like taking the train from the city to the beach. Concrete, traffic, pollution, and then a little less concrete and then a little less traffic and then a little less pollution and then voilà: the vast, undulating blue-green sea.

That was how I tried to hold my first child. As if one day all the arguing and moving about would be over and we would look at each other with the knowledge of all that came before and a deep appreciation for the peace we managed to create. After my separation from his mother, I still hold him that way. As if the cloudy day will pass. As if the distance and lost time will be eclipsed by a newfound togetherness. And it may. But it also may not, and there is very little I can do about it.

Already, months before his birth, I do not hold my second child this way. For starters, I no longer believe in the redemptive power of the calm after the storm. The wreckage on the shore does not disappear because the winds have moved on. When I think of my baby's soon-to-be-born face, full of wonder and unmarred by proximity to rage, I register the value of circum-navigating the storm, of moving inland where it is safe. Even though in the moment it may be more difficult, I now prefer to face the challenge rather than be left with the heartbreaking reality of irreparable damage.

There is also the simple fact that my second child can never be taken from me. We are bound through space and time in the beginningless beginning, that place of infinite mystery. We have met there, on that ground, in a meeting impossible to erase. Even when we are far from each other, we will each possess a fragment of that encounter, buried in the loamy dirt we call our separate selves. I am no longer inexperienced enough to diminish this connection.

There are other things. My stepmother told me a few days ago, again, that she feels I am one of her children, that she raised me as her own. I love her, and yes, in some ways I am one of her children, but in some ways I am not. It may be difficult to ascertain exactly where the line is between the two, but it is beyond question that the line exists. I can decide to care for my stepmother, for instance, but feeling something for my mother, no matter the state of our relationship, is not something about which I have a choice.

I find myself nodding as I read about a study that finds that children living with a stepmother receive a good deal less food, health care, and education than they would if they lived with their biological mother. We're not proud of the way we often preference our biological children, but if we ever want to close the gap, I do think it is something we need to be honest about. I left the conversation with my stepmother thinking, Yes, I would do anything for my first son, within reason. But I would do anything at all for my second child, without reason, without a doubt.

What does that mean for Solomon and me? Is our relationship stained by my confession that our bond isn't the same as the one I have with my biological child? Is it damaged if I say out loud that I love him differently?

I hope not. Solomon will always be my first child. He will forever be the one who inspired me to give endlessly and love selflessly, who showed me that I could become a parent after all. We, too, have a mysterious connection. We appeared in each other's lives when we needed each other the most.

In some ways I saved Solomon's life, and in some ways he saved mine. Without him, my first child, my second child may never have been conceived.

The fetus is now nearly 3 inches from crown to rump and weighs nearly an ounce—about half a banana. Its unique fingerprints are already in place. And when you poke your stomach gently and she feels it, your baby will start rooting— that is, act as if she's searching for a nipple.

June 29

Jesus.

All I can say is thank goodness I am taking the extra dose of meds. Two days ago I checked my e-mail to find a note from my mother threatening to send an attached statement to the editors of Salon.com in response to an interview I did a couple of weeks ago.

In a nutshell, she took offense to a section of my 2001 memoir, *Black, White, and Jewish,* that the interviewer reprinted, in which

I wrote that my parents didn't protect or look out for me, but fed, watered, and encouraged me to grow. In the statement, she called me a liar, a thief (because when I was eight years old I took quarters from her purse during my parents' divorce), and a few other completely discrediting unmentionables. After posting back that unless she wanted out-and-out war, she should rethink her decision to send the letter, I went over to her house to find out what the hell was going on.

Never have I been so frightened by my own mother. She sat me down and called me, in addition to a liar and a thief, "someone who thinks she is a good person but really isn't." She told me that because I wasn't from the South and didn't have the full memory of slavery (read: I am half white), that I don't know what it feels like to be sold down the river, but that's how she felt after reading my book.

For the twenty-five-thousandth time, I apologized for telling my truth in a way that hurt her, and told her that I tried to protect her the best way I knew how. Then I asked whether she thought it was a little strange that I wrote about my struggle in an attempt to get her to take care of me, but here we were talking about how I should be taking care of her. Again.

She grew quite vicious. I told her repeatedly that I didn't think that what she was saying was very maternal. After two hours trying to convince her of the merits of my existence, I left the house shaking.

Glen was extremely upset: This is how she treats you, even when you're pregnant?

Between him and my father, who wrote my mother a letter

saying that as parents it is their job to be proud of my accomplishments rather than undermine my livelihood, I managed to keep it relatively together, but it hasn't been easy.

I keep asking myself, If she's not able to put the needs of the baby first when he's inside of me, how is she going to do that when he's a walking, talking little boy?

June 30

Went with Glen to see his teacher, a high lama from Tibet who escaped by crossing the Himalayas on foot after the Chinese occupiers murdered his father. I always love going to see Khenpo, but given the last few days, it was even more special, like entering another dimension, a surreal world beyond the realm of explanation. He fed us huge beef ribs, the biggest I have ever seen, that he ate with a gigantic knife, expertly paring the meat away from the bone. Then we drank bone soup, which is supposed to be good for physical strength and heating up the body, but which made me want to throw up.

I can barely understand Khenpo when he talks, but Glen gets every word, and the two of them and another lama from Bhutan sat around telling jokes and laughing. I was so tired I had to go into another room to lie down, but I could hear them all the way upstairs and felt comforted, like I was in a pure land and the laughter of the dharma deities was my lullaby.

When we left, I asked Khenpo to bless the baby in my belly. He tapped my stomach and laughed. Bless the baby yourself! At first I was put off, then I realized it was his way of telling me I am as much a deity as he is, and that I shouldn't idealize him and deprecate myself. I have the power to bless my own baby.

July 5

I am at Alta Bates hospital in Berkeley, trying not to freak out. Last night I ate steak and spinach and salad and mint chocolate chip ice cream, and then got an awful pain in my stomach, like someone had taken a knife and stuck it into my gut. When I couldn't take it anymore, I called an ambulance and hobbled downstairs. By the time they got to the building, I was on the sidewalk on my hands and knees, doubled over with pain.

I crawled in the back and told the EMTs my blood type, doctor's name, and that I am four months into a normal pregnancy. The EMT, whom I expected to, I don't know, take my temperature or something, looked at me and said she didn't believe I was actually sick. She said that if I were in as much pain as I said I was, I would be perspiring, or at least breathing heavily, and there were no signs of either, which made her skeptical.

I was like, um, are you kidding me? You think I just wanted to come and get into an ambulance for fun? And then she said, Well, ma'am, are you sure you aren't involved in a domestic dispute? My jaw dropped open almost to Chile. Then she changed course and asked if I had been taking drugs.

Fortunately, Glen drove up behind the ambulance at that moment, and I told the EMT to let me out. Unbelievably, she started saying all of this crazy stuff like they couldn't just let me go, I had to sign something and blah, blah, blah, which seemed absurd, considering she had just told me there was nothing wrong with me.

When we finally arrived at the emergency room, a nice intern checked my vitals and then rolled in a portable ultrasound. After a few seconds of searching, I heard the baby's heartbeat and then the intern say the baby looks fine before bursting into uncontrollable sobs on the gurney. Talk about drama. I had been lying there thinking that I would rather die than lose the baby, and if I had to die to save him, that would be okay.

I didn't have to try to feel that way. There was no ambivalence, no inkling of possible relief at being let off the hook. I knew the truth of this as intimately as I knew my own name: My child must live. Period. End of story. Done.

Dr. Lowen arrived. The pain had subsided a little, and we were all close to letting it go as one of those crazy, bizarre moments in a pregnancy. But just as the intern started to fill out the release form, the pain started again, stronger than ever, and that's when they started talking about a morphine drip for the pain. At that point I would have injected orange juice into my veins if they told me it would stop the pain, but morphine? I had visions of my baby emerging from the womb incoherent and addicted to opiates. As if reading my mind, Dr. Lowen said that it was relatively safe, and that sometimes during pregnancy you have to prioritize the mother's health. I nodded skeptically as the intern injected the needle in my arm.

I was admitted just as I fell into an opium-induced haze, and now here I am, the next morning, with a second IV in my arm and doctors coming in and out trying to figure out what's wrong with me. I keep suggesting to them that it's intestinal. I've been taking those giant iron tablets and eating ridiculous, absurd amounts of food. So far the internist and Dr. Lowen both say that the pain would be lower if it was intestinal.

Whatever it is, I am really happy to have this drip.

July 6

The perinatologist came in today. She said that even though my blood and urine look normal, the location of the pain suggests a possible kidney infection. She recommended a baby-safe antibiotic. I will get it through the IV for the first two days and if the pain decreases, I can take the last dose at home. I asked her three times about the effects of the antibiotics on the baby, and if there were *any* studies that even hinted at adverse effects on the infant. Then I quizzed her on the morphine. She was very nice and assured me that both were okay. Not ideal, but okay. I asked her if she thought it might be intestinal. She didn't think so.

Glen came in just as she was leaving, with big bags of food. I dished it out on my pale green laminated tray, and poured us both some lemonade. I don't know what I would do without him. What do people do without other people? Why is it that so few people are competent in the caretaking department? I feel like the luckiest woman alive to have him sitting with me, going over the details of my conversation with the doctor as if his life depended on it, too.

I am concerned, but I'm also not so into being in the hospital. I have never felt comfortable with using Western medicine exclusively, which explains the small army of healers I have assembled over the years. I am especially not happy with the way the doctors dismiss my opinion of what might be wrong with me. Glen agrees it is hard to have faith in a place where people come in with one thing and then die from something else, but he thinks we should wait and see.

I want to call Marie, the M.D. homeopath, but (a) she's in Alaska, and (b) it might be dangerous to mix the systems. If Marie tells me to take something, then I will have to figure out how it interacts with what I am getting here; if she has a different diagnosis, all of the doctors will be in disagreement, and I will be lying in my hospital bed betwixt and between, not sure what to do. Better to take this train to the end and then try the other if it doesn't kill me.

The only thing that makes staying bearable is the nurse coming in every two hours to check the baby. It's like having my own personal Doppler. I hear his quick little heartbeat, whoosh-whoosh, whoosh-whoosh, several times a day, and into the night.

Fantastic.

July 8

The antibiotic has caused some kind of freak reaction. My white and red blood cell counts have plummeted, ditto for the hemoglobin. I now have acute, medication-induced anemia. The perinatologist came in, scratched her head, and I haven't seen her since. For some unknown reason, an infectious-disease doctor took her place, and she thinks we should discontinue the first baby-safe antibiotic and try a different one. As far as I can tell, there still isn't any indication in my blood tests that I have a kidney infection, but the pain hasn't let up and, well, it seems to be the only thing they can think of.

I asked the infectious-disease person if she thought it could be intestinal and she shook her head. She was very nice, too—slow, methodical, and seemingly knowledgeable. But when I asked her why she, an infectious-disease person, was put on my case, she didn't have a good answer, and that sounded alarm number 9,000.

Glen, exhausted from trying to get a good night's sleep on a coat rack disguised as a daybed, looked over at me after she left and asked what I thought. I said, I think all of these people are crazy and I should call Marie. And then a nurse walked in the door with the new medicine and started hooking it up to the IV.

July 9

Well, I have been here four days and don't have a diagnosis. The pain ebbed slightly today, but when one of the nurses opined that I might not need the morphine drip, I panicked. It hasn't ebbed that much.

I have come to the conclusion that hospitals are not places for healing. The food is awful, the environment depressing, and the constant intrusion of the nurses makes resting almost impossible. I know I should be grateful that I have health care at all and insurance to pay for it, but it's hard when just as I am about to doze off, a nurse comes in to take my vitals.

Glen brought me some scarves to toss around the place, so I climbed out of bed this morning and walked around the room with my IV pole trailing behind me, "decorating." Now my bed has a beautiful pale green cloth over it, and the faded Seurat and Monet prints are all covered with gold and burgundy. I put the lilies Glen brought me on the little table next to the bed, and my books and laptop on the swiveling tabletop I'm using as a desk. Now I am sitting here typing in my favorite sea-green robe with pale pink flowers, and feeling a little more relaxed, like a part of home has been magically transported to the hospital.

A few minutes ago, my father and stepmother called. They were each on different phones in their apartment, asking questions and extracting new information. They're worried and want to know if they should come out. Judy says she can make chicken soup, and my father says he can just sit in the hospital with me. Neither of them can understand why my mother, who lives nearby, hasn't come to see me.

After our last encounter, I can't say I am in a hurry to see her. What I can say is that I have to focus on cultivating relationships with people who have the ability to love me the way I need to be loved.

Not just for my sake, but for the baby's.

July 10

I have got to get out of here. I am getting progressively worse, not better, and when I asked one of the doctors this morning how much this little visit is costing he couldn't say exactly, but somewhere in the ballpark of five to seven thousand dollars a day. Could that explain why there is no real hurry to release me? Is that cynical or savvy?

A little while ago, a hematologist came in and told me he was surprised to see me looking so well because according to my blood counts, I should be close to unconscious. Then he started talking about the point at which we should talk about scheduling a transfusion. Transfusion? Glen and I nodded along with him, but the moment he left I told Glen that it was time to go. I've lost all faith in this place, and I feel strongly that I have to get out while I can. The anemia is acute, but I can treat that at home with beef, spinach, and even iron shots, if necessary. The pain has lessened somewhat, and if I can take two or three Tylenol every few hours, I think I can manage.

Our plan for getting out is to tell each and every doctor and nurse that comes in that I plan to leave tomorrow and that they should either tell me why that isn't possible, or start making preparations for me to leave.

We also called Marie, who said it sounded intestinal, especially in light of the fact that I have been taking the iron capsules (!!!). She instructed me to switch to a liquid diet and get the nurse to give me a laxative.

Glen went to get soup and I put in my request for a laxative, telling the nurse in the same breath that I am going home tomorrow. She said she would contact the doctor about the laxative and that she doubts very much that I will be able to leave tomorrow as there is no indication of it in my chart.

I JUST TALKED to the last doctor that had to be convinced and she finally, reluctantly, said I could leave. Not that I gave her any choice. *I am leaving tomorrow* has been my mantra since ten-thirty this morning, and as of about forty-five minutes ago, when the nurses confirmed that they finally got in touch with my doctors, it seems to be working.

At two o'clock I still wasn't sure. One of the residents came in and told me she wasn't comfortable releasing me because my pain wasn't completely gone and my blood counts were so low. I was like, hello, I agree with you on how upsetting and strange this all is, I just don't agree that staying is going to turn it around because if it was, wouldn't it have already? I stayed calm and didn't say anything because she started talking about giving me an AMA, which Glen explained is a slip that says I have left the hospital "against medical advice." I would have to sign it and clear the hospital of any liability should something happen to me after I leave.

The news that the only thing standing between the hospital and my release is a signature was a tremendous relief, and I was ready to sign right then and there. But after she left, Glen told me that sometimes insurance companies look unfavorably at patients who leave AMA, and could do anything from raise my premium to refuse to continue my insurance at the end of the term. I am aghast but so exhausted and weak that the most I can do is shake my head in disbelief. My will to ask a lot of questions about how that can be legally possible and whether or not most people know this is just gone.

Anyway, I don't want to go on a whole bender against the health-care system. I've been sick in places where there are no doctors and no hospitals, and that was beyond horrendous, but my goodness. It's like the old Gil Scott-Heron song about people walking on the moon while his sister is living in a tenement and getting bitten by rats.

Which brings me back to the matter at hand: Since I replaced the copious amounts of chicken and salad I was eating with soup, my stomach feels a thousand times better. Which is good because a nurse just told me that since I am leaving tomorrow, she is going to pull the morphine to see what happens overnight. I have become so dependent on the drip, I feel like a child being asked to hand over my blanket, pacifier, and favorite stuffed animal right after my mom has left the building. She's in the car, driving away, and the people taking care of me say, Okay, let's just have your blankie and your binky and your little piglet.

The strangest thing is that the doctors and nurses act like it's no big deal, like they're just pulling a sugar-water drip out of my arm and not one of the strongest opiates on the planet. I want to scream out, But I love my little white button! Can't I take it home with me? Which is the closest thing to addiction I've ever felt, if I don't count shoe shopping.

July 12

Home!

My levels are scary, way below normal. I went to see Marie, and she told me to eat boiled chicken, applesauce, something called congee, which is basically rice cooked over and over again until it is total mush, and vegetables overcooked 1950s style. She also told me to rest, and if possible to have people come and take care of me 24/7 for two weeks.

Argh. The idea of people taking care of me 24/7 for fourteen days was hard to wrap my mind around. Who could stop working, parenting, and maintaining their own lives to take care of

December 20

I wrote the baby a note this morning, thinking he might need a little reassurance.

Dearest baby,

Hi, sweetheart. It's time for you to come out of Mommy's stomach. I know it is all cushy and warm in there and you are enjoying all your favorite foods, but I promise you'll like it out here, too. Mommy and Daddy love you and we can't wait to see you and kiss you and take care of you.

Don't be afraid. Mommy hasn't done this before, either, but I know we can do it! We'll do it together.

Love,
Mommy

December 21

I feel as if we have all merged. Glen, the baby, and I have become one unit. I've gone from one to three.

Tonight I feel ready. I give. I surrender. I know it's completely beyond my control.

There is nothing for me to do except let go and let it happen.

Do you hear me, little one? I'm waving the white flag. Do your thing.

I'll be there.

December 22

He's here!

But may I ask one small but very relevant question? Why the hell didn't anyone tell me how much it was going to hurt? The only thing that could ease that pain was an *epidural,* and if I do this again, which at the moment I cannot imagine, I will demand one after the first contraction, if not before.

The whole thing was a miracle, but more on that later. At the moment I must document my newfound respect for every human being that has given birth, and I retract my judgment of every woman who has had or will have a scheduled C-section. Maybe I just have a low threshold for pain, but I don't think so. It is *outrageous.* I remember screaming, somewhere in between the toilet, the birthing pool, the bed, and the shower, that I couldn't believe every person on this earth got here this way. It just doesn't seem possible.

But it is, and now, thirty hours after it all began, I have a little me every hour, seven days a week? Do people even do that any-more in our crazy culture? What, then, do sick people do? They hire caregivers, obviously. But then you're living with a stranger, and I can't think of anything more stressful and depressing. Maybe people can come in shifts? Of course Glen says he can do it all and doesn't need help, but even though I joke about the imaginary cape he wears, he's not Superman.

Marie also told me to visualize a cute, normal, healthy baby, and a healthy remainder of my pregnancy. So that's what I've been doing all afternoon, while making congee and burning three pots of rice in the process.

July 17

I felt a little sorry for myself last night. I've been doing every-thing I am supposed to, but my labs are not improving as dra-matically as they should. I've really taken a hit. Today my hematocrit, which is supposed to be between 36 and 50, is at 27. My hemoglobin is holding at 9. It should be between 12.5 and 17. The only good news is that my white blood cells, which were completely wiped out, are coming back, with a reading today of 9.5, which is perfect.

I refused to let anemia hold me back, though. Today I:

- Watched three episodes of the sixth season of *Sex and the City*. I'm rooting for Miranda and Steve, even though that black Knicks doctor (Blair Underwood) is so sexy and it is nice to finally see an eligible, foxy black man on the show.

- Baked and ate an entire organic marble cake. *Delicious*. I see much baking in my future.
- Forced myself out of the house for a walk around the park. The sky was fiery red and purple, and there were lots of people out walking their dogs and riding bikes. I didn't get far, but it was heavenly to get some air.
- Pitched, to *Salon* and *Slate,* an interview with Spike Lee on his new movie, and did a little work on an essay for an anthology on guilt I agreed to write.

I am tired, but not dead.

July 19

Dinner at my mother's. She invited me with this loving, the-other-day-never-happened e-mail that of course sent me into a tizzy of indecision. What pregnant daughter doesn't want to be close to her mother? There should be a support group: Ambivalents Anonymous.

I asked Glen to come because I was truly, honestly, afraid of being alone with her. The last encounter was that disturbing.

We went over and she was completely angelic, as if a month ago she didn't tell me I was a piece of shit and threaten to ruin the reputation it has taken fifteen years to build. With Glen nearby, I let her feel the baby in my womb, and put her ear to my stomach to hear his little sounds.

It was sort of nice, in a strange, disturbing kind of way. It was sad to notice that I was happier to leave than I was to arrive. I know it sounds crazy, but I kept thinking about Marvin Gaye and how he was killed by his own father.

As a mother-to-be, I feel I have to look at these feelings, no matter how far-fetched they may seem. My protective instinct is way up, and there's no way I am going to ignore it. It is abundantly clear that between my mother and me, I am the only one focusing on what my baby needs.

July 20

Feeling much better today. I woke up with that blissed-out, "I am pregnant woman, hear me roar" vibe. I must really be hitting the second trimester now. I feel the baby so much, his presence like a little glow in my belly. It's way stronger than the quickening of a few weeks ago, that slight, supersubtle whisper of baby consciousness. Instead of the first hello, the first mutual acknowledgment of what exactly is going on here, now it's like a whole conversation between us.

I am having a baby!

For lunch, Glen and I went to the French restaurant around the corner from the apartment. I am really showing now, and people everywhere we go look at me and smile and ask questions. There was a bit of a wait at the restaurant and the couple in front of us gave us their space in line. The woman said she remembered what it was like to be pregnant and hungry in a room full of other people eating.

That is happening more and more, random women starting conversations about the trials and tribulations of pregnancy. I can tell by the way Glen shuts down when they approach that he finds it intrusive and strange, but I like it. It's the first club I've unequivocally belonged to, and I understand tribalism much more as a result. The world really does become divided into the people who know this land and those who don't.

Over lunch Glen and I talked about the amnio, for which I have now missed three appointments. In my opinion, we've already done the pre-amnio blood-test version of the amnio, which came back normal, with no indication of Down's or anything else, so why push it? The amnio would be a follow-up to that, a just-to-make-sure kind of thing, and we'd get to find out boy or girl. Glen says it is up to me. He doesn't believe in a lot of tests, the whole cult of getting everything just because we can, just because it is available. In his opinion, the baby is healthy, and if it's not, we'll deal.

I was into the amnio until I read about the one-in-three-hundred chance of miscarriage. No one I know has ever had a problem, but I just can't get too excited about a huge needle that close to my baby. On the other hand, I have to be honest with myself about being able to care for a baby with special needs. I don't think I can do it. And I definitely want to know ahead of time so that I can make an informed decision. On the third hand, I read that it is not unusual to get a false positive, and then you're really in the wringer.

After we ate, I got really, really tired and came home and went to sleep. I woke up still tired and with that run-down feeling that comes, I think, with a low red blood cell count. Sonam says that even though I am sick, I have to find a way to keep exercising, even if it is just a little. If I feel better tomorrow, I will go for a swim in the morning before I sit down to work.

July 21

Speaking of work. I have no desire to do any. My mind just doesn't have any sparkle, which I find alarming, since my job basically depends on sparkle.

Went to a prenatal appointment at Dr. Lowen's. I mentioned that after the hospital visit I am thinking even more about a home birth. She said, You know, you have to make sure you've got your priorities straight. It's okay to have a baby at home, but a home birth is more for the mother. You go to the hospital for the baby.

My first reaction was anger: How dare she pit me against my baby! If it's better for me, it will be better for the baby. But then I started thinking about the baby, and how wrecked I would be if something went wrong. I remembered my stepmother saying that if something happened to the baby I would never forgive myself. She's right.

Glen is still against a home birth, and when I showed him *The Birth Book,* which Carl and Martine gave me, with all of the amazing pictures of people looking all natural and groovy and organic and healthy, he said, Yes, but they don't put the pictures of home births gone wrong in the book, you don't see those pictures. To which I countered that they don't tell you about the hospital births gone horribly wrong, either. They don't take pictures of all of the C-sectioned moms that could have had natural births. They don't blow up pictures of episiotomies and put them up on the wall next to the cute one-year-olds.

We did another blood test. Dr. Lowen doesn't have any idea why I had the reaction I did to the antibiotics, and isn't quite sure what to make of the fact that my counts aren't back to normal, but she is reassured that now they are going up, and not down.

Me, too.

July 27

I spent a good hour this morning standing in the kitchen in my underwear trying to figure out new and exciting ways to ingest iron-rich molasses. First I tried heating soymilk and dissolving the molasses in it, kind of like a molasses hot chocolate. Barf. Then I tried spreading it like peanut butter on toast. Super barf. Then I tried just sucking on a spoonful. Oh my God, I almost passed out, it was so disgusting.

Solomon arrives in a couple of days for orientation at the new school we decided to send him to here in Berkeley. His mother found an apartment close to the school, and we have agreed that he should live with her primarily, and see me on weekends, and for meals during the week.

I am nervous about the whole arrangement and feeling overwhelmed. I am not going to be able to take care of him as much as I usually do, but I don't want him to feel displaced by the baby. To calm my nerves I made a little schedule that includes a few things I know he'll like. He's old enough to take care of himself a bit, and also be helpful to me. Right?

August 1

Solomon left today. He didn't help, exactly, but I did enjoy hanging out with him. Even though I am ginormous for five months, I can tell the baby thing is a bit abstract to him. I had to keep reminding him that I can't do the things I used to do, like walk up five flights of stairs. Or work all day, go out for dinner, a movie, and then to the bookstore to look at magazines.

Orientation at his new school seemed to go well. He came back with a big smile on his face and several new "friends." He didn't want to hear the lecture I gave him about throwing the word "friend" around with people you hardly know, though. After a few minutes he was like, Okay! Can we go to the burrito place now?

Last night Glen and I talked about the difference between mothering and smothering. Mothering has to do with setting appropriate boundaries and giving kids room to be themselves. Smothering has to do with projecting all of your fears and anxieties onto kids and not giving them a moment's peace. I am determined to do the former and not the latter, but it isn't easy. I notice how much I problematize different aspects of Solomon's identity, calling attention to behaviors that aren't just so and constantly making little corrections. I notice that I want to know his thoughts and feelings a little too much.

I asked Glen about his mother, and what she did right in raising him. She was abandoned as an infant, he said, and ended up graduating from Boston University at a time when very few women, and even fewer African-American women, were able to do so. She was also a single mother at a time when it was socially taboo. She went to graduate school, and then worked as a counselor in a women's prison for twenty-six years.

Tears didn't well up in Glen's eyes, but I could tell he was moved remembering her fortitude. She worked long hours, he

said, but he always had a hot dinner, and never felt that he had to
fend for himself. She created such a strong network of friends that
he always felt he had three or four mothers. She gave him room,
he continued, but she was also clear about her expectations. "I did
well in school," he said, "lettered in three sports, and almost died
of mortification whenever I did something she didn't approve."

She wasn't a saint, he said, but she made some choices to
ensure that he would have a better life. "The most important
thing she did was move us from New York to California, to give
me a chance to grow up without the judgment that came with
being a child born out of wedlock in a community where everyone gossiped." He paused. "She let go of everything she knew,
family, friends, community, to give me an opportunity to live free
of that burden, and looking back now, I'm sure it saved my life."

We kept talking about their relationship. Glen left graduate
school just before getting his master's degree to care for her when
she was ill and then dying of cancer. At one point in the conversation, he said something that he often says when we discuss raising
children and the state of masculinity: "Boys need their mothers."

It wasn't the first time we've talked about his mother and the
decisions she made, but after the last encounter with my own
mother, I can relate a little more to the idea of leaving what is
familiar to create a happy life for your child. I can see the importance of making decisions that enable your child to be not just
physically safe in an environment, but emotionally and psychologically safe as well. If the well-being of my own child doesn't
inspire me to break through my ambivalence about a person or
situation and act more decisively, I have no idea what will.

August 2

I've started swimming. Tonight it was just a teenaged couple and me wading around in the fog. A few nights ago it was me and an older woman who swims every night at nine. Both swims were relaxing. I could see the lights of the city through the steam rising off the pool, and the water was soothing and warm. So far, the baby seems to love being in the water. I imagine he goes right to sleep as I stroke and glide.

On Saturday, I made the mistake of going swimming in the middle of the day, when the pool was overrun with, in my humble opinion, bratty, privileged kids. They bumped into me, swam across my lane, threw footballs over my head, and generally ran around paying no attention to anyone but themselves. I kept standing in the shallow end at the break in my laps so that their mothers would see that I was no ordinary lap swimmer, I was a *pregnant* lap swimmer, damn it. I deserved some modicum of respect, even if just for safety. But the mothers ignored me, too, and kept chatting and glancing approvingly at their kids as they whooped all around me.

The whole time I was thinking about how I will be with the baby, and how he will never be so rude and how I as a parent will never be so checked out. Then I thought, Well, maybe those moms are over there talking about their mastectomies or their husbands' affairs. Maybe this is the first break they've had in weeks. Who knows? They could have been talking about their vacation in Tahiti, but I certainly felt less bitchy toward them when I imagined that they, like everyone else, have problems.

August 4

Glen and I went to have the amnio. We went, even though I was on the fence and even though if there were something wrong it would be too late to do anything about it. "Something wrong" being Down syndrome or worse. "Anything about it" being an abortion.

The receptionist warned me that it would be a three-hour appointment, because in addition to the procedure itself, I would need to undergo routine counseling. She didn't say what kind, and when I asked, she made it sound like preparatory counseling, like you might get before taking an HIV test. How to be prepared for the worst. When we got there, the counseling, which we had to agree to have before they would administer the amnio, turned out to really be "genetic counseling." We were taken into a little room by someone who worked not for the hospital but for a biotech company based in Los Angeles. This very nice woman proceeded to do a "genetic intake" on me and Glen, asking about the race, national origin, and health of family members as far back as we could remember.

The flow from signing in to sitting in the woman's office was so seamless that it took me about ten minutes to realize that something other than what I expected was going on. I was, like I suspect most of the young and middle-aged women in the waiting room, so focused on doing something beneficial for my baby and so excited about seeing him in the ultrasound preceding the amnio that the nice woman could have been asking for rights to my firstborn's stem cells and I wouldn't have noticed.

Glen was less distracted, and as I felt his discomfort I asked the relevance of the information being gathered. I also asked who would own the information, and if my privacy was protected by law. Again, call me paranoid, but I saw the movie *Gattaca*. Genetic discrimination, though not as prevalent today as other forms of discrimination, is not just a paranoid delusion. We don't know what kind of world our children will inherit.

The very nice woman explained that this was a way to screen for potential genetic disorders. She explained that all the information was confidential, and that her computer linked only to the company's database and she had to have a special access code to even turn it on. She explained that the results, my baby's genetic tree, would be shipped to a completely secure facility somewhere in Southern California. She explained that there are, in fact, laws in place that prohibit her company or any other company from using the information for testing, research, or anything else.

I started to feel very uncomfortable. How harmless could it be if it required so much security? It is not too difficult to imagine my son's genes being used against him. If he is predisposed to sickle-cell anemia and heart disease, for example, and potential employers can call this up with a stroke of the keyboard, will this make him less employable? If insurers can call up a family history of diabetes, dementia, or some other disease that is costly to maintain, will they insure him? At what price? These are only two scenarios that gave me pause. I shared them with the very nice woman, and she reminded me about the laws. I reminded her that laws change, you know, and usually to facilitate economic expansion. I can't think of another industry with as much momentum as biotech.

I think she was shocked when I decided against the amnio, but she tried to appear nonjudgmental and supportive. I was a little shocked myself. Amnios are as common as breastfeeding. Even though I was on the fence, I never really thought I'd go through my pregnancy without having one. But what can I say? When she told me that she wasn't sure, exactly, where the fluid was transferred after the test, I lost faith in the whole system. Was I sure I could handle a child with special needs? Absolutely not. Did I feel certain that my baby was going to be more than healthy? Absolutely. Was that anything other than magical thinking? Hard to say.

I did go for the ultrasound, though. To make sure the baby has all ten fingers and toes and both legs and arms, and none of the early signs of other problems. There was also the issue of finding out the sex.

As I lay naked from the waist down on the metal table with cold gel slathered across my belly, a woman who has been doing ultrasounds for thirty years zipped from one side of my baby's face to the other, one hand to the other, one organ to the other. After a few clicks and a few anxious questions from me about whether or not everything looked normal, she asked if we wanted to know if our child was a girl or a boy. I looked at Glen and he said it was up to me. I've never been able to stand someone else knowing something I don't, so I said yes. Well, the technician said, he's definitely a boy. Without a doubt.

A boy!

I knew it.

My boy!

Then she showed us his face and butt and elbow, none of which were the least bit identifiable to me.

As my son squirmed in response to her prodding and poking, at one point turning all the way around to avoid her probe, I wondered aloud if we might be disturbing him with all of our measuring. The woman looked at me with, what can I call it? Disdain? Condescension? I shook my head, trying to meet her halfway, after all, she *had* spent thirty years doing this. I'm just a newbie. That's ridiculous, she said. You're just projecting. And then she roughly wiped a fraction of the gunk off my stomach and told me to wait for the doctor.

It is an understatement to say that I was ready to go home after all this. Maybe I am just hormonally challenged, but as we walked into the bright sun of the parking lot I thought about how fiercely protective I am of this being growing inside of me. That medical office might as well have been a lion on the prowl for fresh kill.

I felt a sense of dread as I wondered about the hundreds of skirmishes before me, and the long and obstinate arm of the culture reaching into my boy's mind and possibly into his very DNA. I clutched Glen's arm more tightly, straining to imagine how I would negotiate it all without his stable presence and fierce intelligence.

Together, we might be able to make it. Alone, I am not so sure.

Five

Oh, that it were possible to write about having a baby in America without writing about not having a baby. I am talking about abortion of course, arguably one of the most controversial medical procedures of our time. As I write, teenagers are taking up collections to travel across state lines to "terminate," and twenty-something women are giving birth to babies they don't want and can't take care of because they think abortion is murder. Right this second, medical students are protesting the ban on teaching them how to perform abortions, and doctors are being stalked and murdered for making abortions available.

In our country, the issue of abortion is used as a litmus test for personal morality and political loyalty, which makes writing about having one dangerous. It doesn't matter that more than one million women have abortions every year, or that you would be hard-pressed to find a family or group of friends in which no one had gone through the ordeal. The moment you talk about abortion publicly, you run the risk of being attacked. Or your story being co-opted and pressed into service.

A few months ago, I was doing research for an article. Amid the 679,000 entries that flashed across my screen, I came across my name in the blog of someone claiming to be a former classmate. He cited a piece I wrote a decade ago on using an abortion as an opportunity to reflect on what life would be like if women were forced to bear children they didn't want. In an attempt to provide a counterpoint to the emotional trauma of abortion, I posited a way to think about the choice as an empowering option that was the result of many years of political struggle.

But the blogger didn't see the piece in this context, and accused me of being "defiantly proud" of having had an abortion, and of "coming close to suggesting that it would be a good thing if all women had abortions." Both of these statements, in my view, were gross misinterpretations, and yet I suppose they were also understandable extrapolations in light of the author's point of view.

Continuing my search, I began to think about approaching actions in terms of their result rather than their "truth." The question was not whether the blogger's statements were "true"— they were not to me but were very much so to him. The question was about the result of his statements. What is the effect of saying that I am proud of having had an abortion, and that I think it would be a good thing for all women to have one?

I ask because when I think about conceiving a child at thirty-four, carrying and giving birth to another human being, I have to revisit the experience of conceiving and not carrying, conceiving and not giving birth to another human being. I have to revisit this because the two are inextricably linked. I have to preface the discussion because it would be easy to distort what I write here and use the distortion as another log on the out-of-control bonfire that is the abortion debate in America.

That is not my intention.

I had an abortion at fourteen, in a little medical office on Geary Street in San Francisco, in what was then called the French Medical Building. It was a foggy San Francisco day and I was wearing pink *Flashdance*-y leg warmers over the calves of my faded jeans. The procedure itself was uneventful. I remember a hideously long needle and then the pain of it piercing my cervix, followed by the whirring of a machine. I remember the doctor, a severe, quiet, older woman with small hands and gray hair. I remember the assistant telling me what was happening, step by step. I remember it being over much more quickly than I anticipated and feeling relief as I walked out of the building and felt the cool San Francisco air against my face.

For years I thought very little about the experience. It was behind me, a choice I made to save my life, a choice I made because there was no other choice. At the time, I lived with my mother in a small apartment in a modest neighborhood. I had just finished the ninth grade. I was headed to a private school that held much promise. I loved my boyfriend, but I was a child, and so was he. Though my boyfriend would second-guess our decision twenty years later, at the time I did not. I added it to the list of experiences that made me who I was at the time: a young woman who had been through a lot. A young woman who was beginning to expect that life would be difficult, complicated, painful.

It wasn't until college that I began to think about the abortion, to reflect on it as a series of moments—the needle, the doctor, the subsequent blocking out of any emotion connected to the event—that lurked in the crevices of my mind, powerfully shaping my self-image. But in college, political necessities took center stage. I was more invested in fighting for the right of women to have abortions than I was in fighting for my right to wade through the aftermath of having my own.

But there was an aftermath, and when I decided I wanted to have a baby, it came flying up at me in the form of a mocking, conspiratorial inner voice. This voice attacked my self-esteem. It challenged the idea that having a baby was something my body could actually do. It said awful things. Things like, The doctor sterilized you, remember? And, Your womb is too damaged now to conceive, let alone carry something as beautiful and important as a baby!

I tried to ignore the voice, to shake it off, but where it had been barely audible before, when I started trying to get pregnant it turned ruthless. In the beginning, I battled it alone, and acknowledged it only when talking to gynecologists. I insisted they convince me I wasn't broken, that having had an abortion did not lower my chance of a successful pregnancy. The doctors looked at me strangely when I pressed them for reassurance. I think it shocked them that I, a "modern woman," would have such fears.

But I did have those fears. Before I became pregnant, they came in the form of the face I sometimes saw in my mind's eye: the Being that hovered. She was a she, with large, dark eyes and an easy laugh. She looked at me, not with anger or blame, but with a quiet sadness. We missed our time, her face said to me. I made it to you but you weren't ready.

I do not regret having the abortion. I regret being lonely and having sex so young, that the Pill was not foolproof, that the permissive culture around me did nothing to prepare me for its consequences. But the abortion itself I do not regret. It is only that I have had to learn to manage the aftermath. First to acknowledge that it exists, and then to reroute it when it appears, to re-lay the cables in my mind so that A no longer connects to E.

Because ultimately, I could not hurl myself into the future and keep a death grip on the past at the same time. I had to wade through the muck, to wake up to the poisonous thoughts I hoarded like jewels. I found that there was a time and a place where I lost faith in my body's ability to sustain new life. There was a time and a place where doubt and shame took the space where hope and confidence should be.

This work of looking, grieving, and reframing didn't take place in a therapist's office, but with Glen, the man I chose to be the father of my child. I told him all of my fears and he held every one, countering what needed to be countered, persevering against all odds to prove me wrong. He told me about abortions he supported women through, and we spoke of the scars that sometimes never heal because the nonpartisan language of healing cannot blossom in a field of polemic.

In these conversations, the mocking voice began to face the inevitability of its defeat. It was silent at first only for a few moments, but then for longer and longer periods until I was pregnant.

The miraculous event shattered its credibility forever.

August 7

Talked with Trajal last night until I couldn't talk anymore. He's going to throw me a baby shower. So sweet. We talked about who should host it with him, where it should be, and how I have to get the registry together. I love the idea of lots of people I like and love welcoming my baby into the world.

Our talking marathon reminded me of college. We used to stay up all night talking about race, gender, art, sexuality, and the latest Madonna video. All while writing papers with titles like "Isolation and Redemption in the Novels of Edith Wharton," "Man as Totem in Abstract Expressionism," and "Sign and Signifier in the Hip-Hop Nation."

Now we're weighing the pros and cons of co-sleepers.

Is this what it means to grow up? I feel exactly the same, just focused on different feelings, images, products, and a little more tired.

I went online this morning and started dealing with the registry. Setting one up means I have to pick some stuff, and that means making decisions. I am especially bananas over the stroller question. Should I get the "travel system" with the car seat that pops between the stroller and the car? The Euro bathtub? *The Happiest Baby on the Block* video?

I was online only for a couple of hours, but I am already feeling overwhelmed by the pregnancy industry. Those marketers just reach right in and get us first-time moms because we don't have a clue what we'll really need. I know that I feel so much anxiety about being ill prepared emotionally and psychologically that I'll buy anything and everything to soothe my jangled first-timer nerves.

On that front, I have embarked upon the massage aspect of my pregnancy. I found a great massage therapist who does this out-of-control prenatal thing with pillows and heating pads and sandalwood oil. I just lie there like a beached whale being slathered and rubbed and relieved of aches and pains I didn't even know I had. It was heaven to surrender to the dimly lit room, Japanese flute music, and tiny dendrobiums in porcelain vases. Of course I had to ask him if he had kids. He said, Oh yes, and my wife insisted I massage her like this every day when she was pregnant.

Lucky, lucky, woman.

August 8

Got a call today from the "genetic counselor"! She thinks that perhaps I have G-6-pd deficiency, a genetic blood disorder that makes all sulfa antibiotics practically lethal, along with random foods like fava beans. She said that may be why I had the reaction in the hospital. It may also explain why I got so sick many years ago in Egypt: I was eating fava beans every single day.

Go figure. The woman I thought was Satan may have just given me my genetic key. If she's right, knowing that I have this disorder could save my life.

Also got an interesting request from a magazine to interview Arthur Miller. I said yes, but after thinking about it, I think I'd rather interview Rebecca, his daughter. I remain interested in the children who manage to emerge from the shadow of well-known parentage. So few make it. Then there's the sobering truth that no matter what you go through, it's like being the poor little rich kid: People just think you're whining. No one wants to hear that adults who grew up in a rarefied world have serious issues. They just don't. You're supposed to shut up and take your last name to the bank.

There ought to be a how-to book for parents in the public eye on how to raise sane, happy kids. I hope one day to be able to write it.

August 9

I have started to look at thin women with something akin to envy. I feel so huge, so invisible in my unfashionableness. This morning I caught myself clocking the straight-leg jeans of a woman in front of me, the pointy little shoes, the body-fitting top. I had never noticed how thin these put-together young

women are. How thin I guess I used to be, how young and unaf-
fected.

Now I am awkward and wide, puffy where I used to be
angular. At my last appointment with Dr. Lowen, I weighed
165 pounds. That's thirty-five pounds gained, and I'm only in
the fifth month. When the nurse's eyes widened, I said, Hey,
what can I say, he's healthy and robust, remember? He likes
to eat.

But it's more than the weight gain, it's the sense of not being
able to turn back. I won't ever be as young as that young woman
again. I may be that thin, though I can't quite imagine it, but I
will never again be that pristine, totally willful young woman.
This descent into powerlessness, and being at the whim of a force
so much stronger than me, has changed me forever.

I always thought I would appreciate not being the object of
penetrating stares and appraisals, but somehow I don't exactly. In
our culture, sexuality is always the subtext, and it feels strange to
be excluded from the conversation.

August 10

Have I documented how much this child inside of me likes
salad? Oh my God! I could eat ten huge bowls a day and it
wouldn't be enough. He also likes black-cherry soda and huge
beef hot dogs with sauerkraut and mustard that give me the most
wicked heartburn.

Glen introduced me to Tums last night at one a.m., when I
couldn't take it anymore and begged him to make it stop. I
thought my esophagus was going to catch fire. Yet another gift

from the little one: heartburn. I wake up in the middle of the night burping and gulping for air.

Attractive.

August 13

I have officially entered into the heated immunization debate. My friend Chaya told me today that she believes that kids are "altered" after being vaccinated, and that I should do everything in my power to prevent the baby from getting his shots for at least the first year. She says before that, their immune systems are weakened because they haven't had enough time to develop, and this creates all kinds of problems. Their emotional affect is often dampened, and, according to her, there is even a correlation between the vaccines and ADD.

I intuitively agree that shooting a newborn up with a huge dose of a deadly disease (or five or six) seems a bit demented, and yet there are millions of people who have been immunized and are just fine. Heck, I was immunized. But still, I'd prefer not to give him a shot of any kind at birth and for at least six months to a year after. And I don't really see the need to give him a vaccine for a disease that's been eradicated.

There was just enough of the religious in Chaya's voice to give me pause, however. When she gave me the name of a friend of hers who has researched the subject exhaustively, I put it in my book with all the other cards with people's names that I've been given over the last five months. When I got home I started looking for guidance from what Glen calls my other husband, the Internet.

I was a bit shocked to find this statement from Dr. Jane Ori-
ent of the Association of American Physicians and Surgeons:

> Measles, mumps, rubella, hepatitis B, and a whole
> panoply of childhood diseases are a far less serious threat
> than having a fraction (say 10%) of a generation afflicted
> with learning disability and/or uncontrollable aggressive
> behavior because of an impassioned crusade for universal
> vaccination.

On the other hand, Children's Hospital of Philadelphia
posted this on its site:

> Vaccines are considered the best way to protect your
> child against diseases that could cause liver damage, liver
> cancer, suffocation, meningitis, pneumonia, paralysis,
> lockjaw, seizures, brain damage, deafness, blindness,
> mental retardation, learning disabilities, birth defects,
> encephalitis or death.
>
> Vaccines are considered by some to be a civic duty
> because they create "herd immunity." This means that
> when most of the people in a community are immunized,
> there is less opportunity for a disease to enter the
> community and make people sick. Because there are
> members of our society that are too young, too weak, or
> otherwise unable to receive vaccines for medical reasons,
> they rely on "herd immunity" to keep them well.

When I talked to Glen about it, we came up with the scenario
of our great-great-grandkids' deciding against vaccinating their

kids against cancer because they hadn't experienced people dying from the disease, and couldn't imagine that there could be a resurgence.

We talked about the risk of driving cars, flying in airplanes, swimming in the ocean. If there was a vaccine developed for HIV or cancer, would we get it, knowing there was a one-in-a-million risk of something going wrong? Probably. We talked about how much we travel. Just a few months before I got pregnant, we flew halfway around the world and passed through six different airports. Even if a disease was eradicated in our country, with so much international exposure, wouldn't it be irresponsible to leave our child vulnerable to contracting it in another country?

But what if our son died at two and a half, after a hepatitis B shot? Or of sudden infant death syndrome the night after being vaccinated? Or developed a learning disability that was later linked to a vaccine?

We talked for hours and at the end of it, I was practically in tears. The magnitude of the decisions, my God, does it ever stop?

August 18

Picked my father up from the airport this afternoon and convinced him to rent a huge SUV to help me bring some things up to the house in Mendocino.

It hit me on the line at Hertz: I am almost thirty-five years old and my father is still helping me move my stuff. I remembered the long drive to New Haven on the first day of college. The car was overflowing with clothes and posters and bedding. At the end of the year, he picked me up from an old, funky house I had moved into, fleeing the dorms. I had thrown everything I owned into black garbage bags that he dutifully slung into the back of the Volvo. I thought of him doing the same for my brother and sister, and how endless it must have seemed to him all those years.

Parenting. Again, I have to wonder, does it ever stop?

He told me that I look good, but tired. He said he wanted to come out to support me because he's been worried and knows how difficult my pregnancy has been. I started to cry. It *has* been hard. My tendency is to think about how much worse other people have it, but the truth is, none of this has been easy.

August 19

A whole gang of us went out tonight to do a reading at Borders from *What Makes a Man*. The essayists who read were funny and moving. I did what I seem to do best these days: beamed and rubbed my big belly.

My father's presence is stirring up old feelings. When I lived in California as a young person, he came to visit only once, when I graduated from high school. I flubbed my valedictorian speech because I was so nervous about my parents being in the same space, breathing the same air. Having him here makes me realize how much I longed for him. We were so close and then suddenly, when my parents moved to opposite ends of the country after their divorce, we were far, and I felt disconnected and lost.

Having him here, playing the father role, feels good and right, archetypally correct. He picked me up today, and we went for a walk around the lake in Tilden Park. On the way home, we stopped at the supermarket for preparatory diapers and baby food. He insisted on paying here, in California, the way he always does there, in New York, which made me smile. I don't know if I can describe it, really. But to see him in the grocery store that I go to every few days, looking at the same checkout people under the same fluorescent lights made me feel more integrated, like my life is finally becoming seamless rather than patched together.

It seems right that the baby is the catalyst for this healing. So far he's been the catalyst for so much that is good in my life. Becoming more patient and less argumentative, learning to be a more accepting partner, even eating more salad!

August 20

I am huge. Just fucking ginormous. Whose body is this, anyway? How big can I actually get? Most days I feel like a sensual Amazon of fertility, but sometimes I am just not up to lugging it all around. Part of it is that my counts are still so low. The anemia is making normal activities downright Herculean. This morning it was all I could do to wash a load of clothes, scramble some eggs, and answer a few e-mails. Then I had to take a nap.

My father picked me up in the afternoon in the big boat of a car that he hates driving, but which I love being driven in. It's my size. We went to see *The Manchurian Candidate,* which was a fascinating look at contemporary masculinity. It was a good example of how mothers often participate in the making of a self-sacrificing, money-and-power-at-all-costs, man-a-tron. They shape the boy into a version of the powerful figure they wish they could be; they shape the boy into a version of the husband they wish they had; they shape the boy into someone who is, in ways barely perceptible to the untrained eye, utterly under their control.

I don't want to be like that.

August 25

My father and I had a long talk today about my determination to be happy. The truth is that I am happier now than I have ever been, and I am amazed by how much that has to do with falling in love with this baby inside of me.

As a child of divorce, it has been hard for me to grasp the concept of a functional family dynamic. What does it look like? How does it make you feel? I'm so used to equating family with conflict and psychological wounding, unbridled jealousy and simmering rage, that I've been unknowingly re-creating it in every major relationship I've had.

The pain of those relationships should have been motivation enough to change, but it has taken the desire for my baby to have a different experience to drive me to make different choices. In my role as fearless protector, I have become more decisive and self-aware, less prone to being yanked about by the needs and wants of others. I'm not sure how it happened, but it seems that in being able to love my child unconditionally, I am more able to love myself unconditionally, which means putting up with a lot less bullshit from others.

It's so cliché and remedial, but I think this pregnancy is teaching me that love is about listening to the people you love, and giving them not what you think they should have, but what they say they need. Love is not about endless negotiation, and recovering from blows landed in the throes of anger, but eliminating those fits completely. Family does not have to be a battleground.

The further along I get in this pregnancy journey, the more I realize that my longing for a child was a longing for an opportunity to try it all again. It was a longing to do family better, to do it right. To create happiness not just for my babies, but for me.

August 27

Back from Mendocino, and my father and I are both exhausted from the drive. Productive visit, though.

Before we left, I showed him all of the little changes and upgrades I've made to the place in preparation for the baby. He was underwhelmed by the two-and-a-half-hour drive, and not convinced I should keep pouring money into a house that my mother could, on a whim, ask me to leave.

He's got a point.

August 29

My father left this morning. I cried walking him to the car and made him promise to come back next year. He said of course, he'd have to come spend time with his grandson. It was hard to see him go, but a relief to have Glen's arms to rest in after he was gone.

Sonam came over in the afternoon. We did our usual Doppler and dipstick dance and then talked about doulas, birth assistants who reportedly ensure shorter labors with less of a chance of a C-section or episiotomy. Since I'm revising my birth plan to include Glen's wishes in the scenario, the doula has emerged as a mutually agreeable possibility. She would massage me during labor, and bring me yummy things, and remind me to turn over or try a new position.

Every time I bring up a postpartum doula, though, someone who can wash clothes and cook food for the first two weeks we're home, Glen shakes his head. We'll be fine, he says. Neither of us wants a stranger so deeply embedded in our intimacy, but I can't imagine how I will feel after I give birth. What if I can't get out of bed, or I am less than functional mentally? Glen pats my hand. You were made for this, he says, look how beautifully you're carrying our baby.

That's easy for him to say, I think. But I do feel better after he says it.

September 2

Today I wandered around San Francisco in the neighborhood where I lived as a teenager. I walked up the hill to St. Mary's Cathedral, down through the housing complex with fountains running through it, and past the concrete bench where I sat my first boyfriend down twenty years ago to tell him I was pregnant. I rubbed my belly and talked to the baby the whole way, showing him where I used to live, and where I used to roller-skate, and where I caught the 38 Geary bus to go to school.

I was amazed by how little has changed. We are so used to thinking that everything revolves around us, that the objects in our world are there because we are, and that without us, they wouldn't exist. I realized today how untrue that is, how thousands passed through the same set of buildings, streets, walkways.

I had the sense of being outside of time. Of watching the world stand still while I moved through it. I was born, I live, and I will die, but the sky goes nowhere.

The thoughts could have been disconcerting, but instead I felt liberated. I felt light walking those hills, watching the memories come up and fade away. I finally understand what people mean when they say that everything changes but everything also stays the same. Life happens where those two meet.

September 8

Glen did a teaching at a dharma center in Marin last night, so we drove across the bridge and took the windy road along the Pacific. The center was beautiful, with an organic farm and lovely Japanese-style buildings. I enjoyed the serenity of the place, and the quiet orderliness of the monastic setting. The food was amazing.

I think I was a shock to some of the monastics, waddling around with my big belly. It amazes me that so many people in America think that in order to be Buddhist you must be a monk or nun. They don't know about laypeople and householders; they don't realize that the dharma can be inflected in just about any lifestyle.

The ride home was long and dark. We listened to Carole

King and Al Green, and the baby kicked up a storm and demanded that we stop and get a Mounds bar.

This morning I got an e-mail from my mother. She received the invitation to the baby shower in New York and wants to throw me a tea at her house in Berkeley on my birthday in November. It sounds reasonable, but also not. Even though a part of me wants to believe that it isn't a setup of some kind, the other part is hesitant.

Against my better judgment, I wrote back that it sounds like a great idea, and I am happy she wants to welcome the baby into her community.

Then I got a really bad headache.

September 12

Interviewed the first potential doula today, Ocean. I liked her until she asked why I'm not having the baby at home. I patiently explained that Glen isn't comfortable with it, and we both want the reassurance of being in the hospital in case something goes wrong. She said that I shouldn't let anyone keep me from the birth experience I want, and I had to explain to her that the birth of my child was not only my experience, but Glen's and the baby's, too. In order for me to have the experience I want, they have to be happy, not just me. Considering the hell I gave Glen on this point, I couldn't believe the words coming out of my mouth. But there they were, and they were true.

Then she asked if I am having the baby at the hospital because I am afraid. And I said, Look, hon, no offense, but I've thought about all of this quite a bit. My decisions are hard-won and

I have no desire to have them questioned by someone I met ten minutes ago.

Is it me, or the hormones?

Needless to say, she's not the right person. She may have meant well, but you simply cannot be an advocate for someone and at the same time think you know more about their wants and needs than they do. It's impossible.

I took a long shower after she left and then massaged my belly with magic anti–stretch mark potion number 59.

My blood counts are creeping toward normal. Still low, but definitely getting better.

September 14

Today I ran into a tree. I have gotten so clumsy. This belly gets in the way of seeing more than two inches in front of me, and my sense of balance is completely shot. I went to go look at the hospital and parked around the corner from the emergency lot we would use on the big day. I got out of the car and walked around to the meter, and as I was scooping quarters from the bottom of my purse, *bam!* I smacked my head into a thick branch and almost passed out.

The hospital was okay. The neighborhood is a bit sketchy compared to the hospital near the house, which is tucked away and surrounded by trees. This one is on a big city street with a lot of empty storefronts and homeless people wandering around. The patients are mostly Mexican, Ecuadoran, and Samoan, and the nursing staff, from what I could see, is largely Filipino.

I met Sonam in the Labor and Delivery ward, and she showed

me the birthing pool and the room where I will labor. It is very large, with hardwood floors and warm, nonfluorescent light. There are two big windows. It wasn't my living room, but it was nicer than most hospital rooms I've seen. It didn't feel institutional. There were no pale green or gray walls, no cold, polished concrete floors.

I was talking to Sonam and the nurses at the nursing station when a woman in one of the rooms started sobbing and screaming, It hurts! It hurts! over and over again. It was the first time I have heard a woman in active labor, and all I could think was: *Drugs!* I want as natural a birth as possible, but I am no masochist. I want that epidural standing by. And that's what I told Sonam in no uncertain terms as I clutched her arm while waiting for the elevator. Make sure we have an epidural close by. When she smiled, I was like, No, Sonam, you don't understand, I am serious.

She said okay.

I said it again as the elevator doors were closing.

Don't forget the epidural!

September 15

I went to see the osteopath today. He's been working on me for years, helping to manage a repetitive strain injury I have that makes writing difficult. He also tends to the aftereffects of a motorcycle accident I had as a teenager, when I thought I could drive a motorcycle around a semi-developed island in a bikini and flip-flops.

He was excited about the baby and told me about all the pregnant women he's treated. When I asked if he had children, he said that he and his first wife had been pregnant, but the baby died at birth from Listeria, a bacterium found in uncooked beef and poultry, and processed foods like hot dogs and deli meats that aren't cooked properly before packaging.

Uch! The heartache. To carry a baby to term and give birth only to have the baby die in the first minutes of life is unbearable to imagine, and yet this happens all over the world, every day. When I told him how sorry I was, he nodded and told me about his second wife and her daughter, with whom he is very close.

My osteopath is such a gentle guy, such a healer. He's so deserving of all kinds of love. He must have been devastated. I stayed cool and kept a good boundary, but really I wanted to get off the table and give him a big hug.

Now that I'm listening, it seems everyone has a birth story, or an almost birth story.

Six

To be put under the heading "What on Earth Was I Thinking?": I first tried to get pregnant while in a passionate relationship with a beautiful, brilliant, and ultimately unfaithful musician. On the road in Tokyo, Århus, Milan, Santa Fe, and other even more exotic climes, the two of us talked about making a baby. Inevitably, the discussion took place in hotel bathrooms—an elegant white marble cube in Bern, a humble ventilated box in North Carolina, a padded art deco creation in Chicago—and on the tour bus, especially after a gig at which a good-looking man had been spotted. A good-looking man who had the requisite physique and the even more requisite over-the-top adoration/obsession for my rock-star girlfriend.

We'd be sprawled on the filthy sofas at the back of the bus at three a.m., still riding the adrenaline from the show and trying not to inhale the exhaust seeping in from the back of the old

Prevo. Undoubtedly she, the girlfriend, would have put a movie
into the DVD player, something like *Hair, Dumb and Dumber,* or
Amadeus. If the band hadn't inhaled it all, we'd be munching on
the remains of food listed on her craft-service rider: carrot sticks
and hummus, a glass of soymilk. If the band had finished everything, I'd be trying to make a meal out of a bag of cashews scored
the previous day at Whole Foods.

During lulls in the action, I would say something like: M
would be good. And she would say, Yeah, we should put him on
the list. Or, I don't know—he's too goofy. Or, He's not that smart.
Or, He's got a great body. Or, He's got a girlfriend who would
never, ever let him do it.

We talked in terms of genetic preferences and of men who
could be fathers but not intrude on our life. We talked of sperm
banks and daddy donors and lifetime parenting partners and
new family configurations. When our straight friends had kids,
we oohed and aahed and declared ourselves godparents, and
when our gay friends had kids, we mined them for details.
Would the child be close to the other biological parent? Did the
donor want involvement? Did it complicate the "primary" relationship?

It was decided that because I wanted the baby most, and
because she had already given birth to one child, I would be the
one to conceive. She would be my coach, protector, cook. She
would also be responsible for naming the baby because I am
awful at naming. And because she was crazy for outrageous biblical names like Hezekiah and Ezekiel, and I didn't have the
energy to resist.

Over a couple of years, we amassed quite a list of willing participants, though I am not completely sure why they were willing. Was it the prospect of being a father sans the daily work of parenthood? The promise of free concert tickets for life? Whatever the reason, when all was said and done, it came down to two men who weren't on our list, two men we knew and loved, two men who were already like family. And so, acting as if our relationship was far more stable and full of fidelity than it actually—I found out later—was, my girlfriend and I masked our nervousness with jocular banter and popped the question.

The proposal went something like this: How would you like to have a baby with us? We've thought about it, and, well, you're one of the only people in the world we can imagine doing this with. Sure, we'd like you to be involved because children need fathers, but you could choose your involvement level. Oh, and we want to get pregnant the natural way, no turkey basters. Is that all right with you?

When we initially proposed, the man I favored immediately took himself out of the running. He had been privy to too many of our conversations in which we reduced men to their genetic attributes. He declared that our relationship was intimate enough, thank you very much. Besides, he said with a Cheshire grin, he didn't know where things might go if we started having sex. I laughed when he said this, and stole a look at his strong, beautiful hands. I didn't disagree.

Our second choice was a man who had been close to my girlfriend for many years in several capacities. John was loyal, kind, and intelligent. He picked us up from the airport. He counseled the girlfriend through each of her several dozen career crises. He had already taken on the responsibility of fathering two children

who were not his own, and one of them had just been accepted to
Harvard. John was also an athlete, an attribute I found particularly alluring. By the time we proposed, he had come to rest in
the position of brother, or, at the very least, lifelong friend.

I liked John.

We asked John in a more gradual way, over time, using the
same questions and phrases, but spaced over months and inter-
laced with conversations about travel, business, and politics. We
asked him to father our child in the way his thoughtful and
methodical personality demanded: with gravity, sensitivity, and as
much tact as we could muster. Because he was already so embedded in our lives, the proposition was not as much about having a
baby as it was about extending our life together and building a
nontraditional but committed family.

We talked seriously about moving to Europe, where the girlfriend had a big following, and where I could write and be cared
for by the thriving holistic midwifery and healing network. I
could learn French, and the baby could be bilingual, and we
could live in one of those charming villages in Switzerland in the
crook of a mountain road overlooking Lake Geneva, a few miles
from the Evian spring. Or we could move to South Africa, where
the girlfriend had a big following, and where we could be surrounded by black people deep in the inspirational throes of the
project of self-determination. John could be our business manager. John could be our husband.

John was not opposed to the idea, or should I say the fantasy,
but this is where it began to get messy. In addition to having
dreams of his own of living in Cuba, he was not altogether sure
that he wanted to enter our relationship. For one thing, the girl-

friend and I fought a lot, and for another thing, John had his own idealistic visions of family, and these visions did not necessarily include two additional women, no matter how dynamic.

There was also the not-minor hindrance of his girlfriend, a woman he'd known since high school and had been involved with for several months. During our discussions, we were surprised to find out that John liked this woman a great deal, that is, when he wasn't talking to us about not liking her and not knowing how to get out of the relationship.

And so it was in the very familiar soup of ambivalence and ambiguity that we began our crazy, rather irresponsible, and beautiful science experiment of trying to make a baby with John. The project included serious and somber conversations at restaurants on the Upper West Side of Manhattan, restaurants that were organic, intercultural, and macrobiotic, restaurants that were futuristic stabs at the kind of hybridity we were, ourselves, considering. Seated around tables with chopsticks and carrot juice and brown rice and Chino-Cuban arroz con pollo, we said, Yes, we want to do this; yes, we think this could be a good thing; yes, why not? We love each other, we are already family, right?

Which led to an evening at one of the hotels we liked, a hotel that felt like home not just because the staff gave us a good rate (fans of the girlfriend), but because we had lived there one summer in a beautiful beige-and-white room that overlooked Broadway and the gorgeous old apartment buildings that line it. I don't remember much of the encounter, only that I concentrated very hard on getting pregnant. And that the next morning I crawled out from under John's heavy limbs and made my way to the bathroom. Steadying myself amid the brushed aluminum and stylized black-and-white prints of orchids, I looked at myself in the mirror and wondered: Is this the face of a pregnant woman? Then I stumbled into an armchair and scribbled a few lines in my journal.

Since accompanying my girlfriend on the road, I used my journal to keep track of our comings and goings. On the inside covers of dime-store notebooks, I made long lists of cities and dates, and pressed my marked-up backstage passes onto the blank sheets in between. I felt that unless I did this, recorded places and times and some tiny sliver, even if only a sentence, there would be no record of the life streaming through each day. And because I am fundamentally a woman who wants stability, I wanted—no, needed—a record, a way to evoke forever the musicians and fans, the airplane flights and bus trips, the hotel rooms and especially the freak encounters that make life on the road, for all of its drudgery, magical.

(An evening in the aforementioned Swiss village, in an alpine chalet overlooking Lake Geneva, comes to mind. Claude, the legend behind the Montreux Jazz Festival, pulling tapes from his archives and there, in his screening room, Aretha Franklin, twenty years ago, playing the piano and singing her heart out.)

Because these elements were such an integral part of our life, they *were* our life, and because I could not imagine that my girlfriend and I would no longer have this life together, I was forced to think pragmatically about bringing the baby on the road. I had moved around a lot as a child and could romanticize the time on the bus as a nomadic lifestyle full of change and diversity. But did I want my child to have rootlessness as an organizing principle? The girlfriend deemed it possible, but I had major doubts, and my scrawled notes from that morning reflected those doubts. After the date and the city and the evening's activity, I scrawled, Baby on the bus? Nursing on the back of a stinky Prevo?

I cannot swear that the way I remember the rest of this story is exactly the way it played out, but I guarantee that only small details may be inaccurate and not the gist of the thing, not the core event. There were days of thinking I might be pregnant. Days of waiting and nights of lying in bed trying to figure out how I was going to explain the how of this baby to my extended family and even, to the extent that it was interested, to the world at large.

At the onset of these days—I would say on day two or three—came the news that John and his girlfriend were no longer seeing each other. Around day seven came the news that John was seeing his girlfriend again, but only to process the breakup and/or talk about the possibility of being together in the future. On day fourteen or fifteen, John came to us and told us that the girlfriend, whom he was now not seeing, was pregnant, and even though he wasn't sure he wanted the baby, he wasn't sure he could stop her from having it.

My girlfriend and I were horrified. Outraged. Deeply hurt. There were long, cross-country arguments on cell phones, and immature, hyperbolic disavowals in doorways. I, for one, was never so happy and relieved to get my period, an event that, from my perspective, took everything down a notch, or ten. Months passed. I stopped feeling like I had lost a popularity contest. I stopped feeling like I had lost a fertility contest. Though my girlfriend was devastated and vowed it would never be the same, the family slowly reconvened. We decided to befriend the actual mom-to-be, and even though I am pretty sure we both secretly fantasized she was carrying a baby that would ultimately belong to us, we came to terms with what in private we labeled John's gullibility.

Which is how I came to be holding John's baby and not my own at a restaurant in TriBeCa ten months later. The birth had been traumatic, and this was one of the first days out of the house for mother and son. We were doing a group dinner, the kind the girlfriend and I did a lot as a way of keeping the extended tribe together. We invited John and his girlfriend/not girlfriend and their baby as a way of saying we still love you, there is room in the fold even though you lied to us, or didn't, and even though you chose someone else over us, or didn't.

It was an extraordinary experience—heartbreaking, really—to be eating fish with one hand, and holding in the other a tiny, beautiful creature who should have been mine, could have been mine, but wasn't.

I will never forget it.

September 18

We've arrived in Miami for the Dalai Lama's teaching: World Peace Through Inner Peace. Glen's teacher sponsored the teaching, and we are here as special invited guests, which means attending various gatherings with His Holiness and various dignitaries from all over the world. The first teaching is tomorrow at eight a.m. Khenpo expects close to twenty thousand people to attend, which is amazing because the television is full of hurricane warnings and evacuation notices. Two days ago there was talk of evacuating Miami, but Khenpo held firm. When we asked why he didn't leave, he said that only the people who are afraid of dying are leaving. And then he laughed his huge laugh. When we landed, the sky was blue, not a cloud in sight.

We checked into our hotel last night and I've been luxuriating ever since. They say the architecture is "Mediterranean Revival," but it's more Moorish Italianate to me. Whatever you call it, it's just stunning, with elaborate tile work and impossibly high ceilings. I just came from a nighttime swim in possibly the most amazing pool ever. It's billed as the biggest in the continental United States, and at 700,000 gallons, I believe it. I swam by moonlight with soft jazz playing and palm trees blowing in the breeze. The hotel was built in the twenties and I truly felt I was in a different era, and the flappers were going to come out and put on a show.

As I swam, I imagined that the water was precious purifying nectar, cleansing my mind and body of thoughts of anger, jealousy, and greed. I thought about how there is no new water, and that all of the water on the planet has been here, cycling through its various incarnations, for millions of years. I thought about how that same ancient water is inside of me, and so part of me has also been here for millions of years.

After a while, I flipped onto my back and looked out into the vast night sky. Floating, I wondered about the baby. Where did he come from? How did he get here? Where will he go?

How is it possible that I love him so much?

September 19

Today was the luncheon with His Holiness. He entered the room with his entourage of attendants and bodyguards, bowing and making eye contact with as many people as possible. The electricity in the room was palpable, like it must have been when Kennedy walked into a room, or Gandhi. When he reached the podium, he paused, looked out at everyone, and said that human beings have different hair and different eye color, we wear different clothes and come from different places. But really, he said, at the fundamental level, we are all the same.

I can't do justice to the moment, but it was amazing, an empowerment. For a brief second, and forever after for some, you could actually feel the truth of what he was saying. It wasn't just a social or political idea, but an actual experience of sameness and, ultimately, of a world not chopped up by dualistic thinking.

It was like the sky opened up.

September 20

Tonight after the teachings, we had dinner in the hotel restaurant. A harried mom with baby in tow spotted my huge, unmistakably pregnant belly, and proceeded to tell me her whole story: the difficult pregnancy, the complicated birth, the intense sleep-deprivation. I smiled through the whole litany and then asked her, But is it worth it? And she looked at me like I was crazy. Oh, of course. It's so totally worth it. You won't believe it. It's like no love you've ever known.

I rest my case.

After my late-night swim, I came back to the room and admired myself in the mirror. I am really getting into my pregnant body. I've finally got the full breasts I've always wanted, and my thighs, which I've always considered just a tad larger than ideal, are now in perfect proportion.

As I was standing there, thinking how downright voluptuous I am, Glen came up behind me and shared a sentiment that won him the Best Thing Your Partner Can Say When You Are Pregnant Award. He said, You've never been more beautiful. Which turned me right then and there into a goddess. I felt so powerful, having just bathed in the moonlight, and rubbed some kind of outrageous-smelling Tahitian oil all over my belly, that I had to turn around and give him the biggest, juiciest kiss ever.

September 21

Landed at JFK and was practically blinded by the newspaper headlines: "Yes She Is!" and "Pregnant and Still Thin." Apparently, a TV star presumed heterosexual is in love with a woman, and most of the rich, pregnant women in New York are starving themselves so that they can stay CWP—cute while pregnant. Both headlines had me at hello. I had to stop at Hudson News.

The pregnancy article is horrifying. It seems that women don't want to wear maternity clothes or lose their waistlines, so they restrict their diets and try to subsist on a bottle of water and an apple a day. I guess they're not having the renaissance of self-love brought on by baby love I'm having. Yikes. The whole idea of DWP, dieting while pregnant, makes me sad and *hungry*.

September 23

Last night I told everybody I am thinking about naming the baby Tenzin. My stepmother looked up from her plate and said, Tenzin? What kind of name is that? Then my father said that no matter what I named him, he was going to exercise his right as a grandfather to call him whatever he wanted, which was Chaim. I told them that Tenzin is the Dalai Lama's name and that I can't think of anyone better to be named after. To which my stepmother responded, Isn't there anyone in the family you could name him after? And my father said, Yeah Rebec, what about Samuel? David? Moishe?

I felt like Judas.

Before we arrived at the question of what to name the first biological grandchild of the Leventhal clan, we focused our collective energy on whether or not my sister, an aspiring actress, should take a role on a reality show. My brother and I were vehemently opposed and got so unbelievably vocal about the whole thing, with my father chiming in from the sidelines with a "legal perspective" and my stepmother picking at her miso cod and trying not to get involved, that my sister finally had no choice but to accuse us of trying to control her life. She stormed out of the room as I yelled, We are only telling you this because we love you, to which everyone nodded approvingly and my father said, That's right, Rebec, after which my sister slammed her bedroom door.

It was my first dinner with them as a ravenous, two-headed, big-bellied omnivore. My father got a huge kick out of watching me eat two California rolls, one filet mignon yakitori, a giant salad, an order of Agadashi tofu, two bowls of miso soup, and an entire order of steamed vegetable dumplings. He kept beaming and saying things like, So you're eating for two, my Rebecca? Eat plenty for my grandson in there, the little schmutzky, and asking if I wanted the rest of his chicken-and-vegetable dish.

September 25

We went to my stepmother's best friend Ronnie's house to break the fast for the Jewish holiday of atonement, Yom Kippur.

Jason, Ronnie's black, white, and Jewish son, with whom I used to watch *The Love Boat* and *Fantasy Island* sprawled on his mom's bed, was there with his new girlfriend. She's Cuban, but has never been to Cuba. Of course this possibility didn't occur to me until after I had talked about how beautiful the island is and how the people are so incredible. The blank look on her face tipped me off. Then I started obsessing about how her family must have lost everything in the revolution and they probably hate Fidel or at least have serious and legitimate gripes. Then here I come, a spoiled American, talking about it like just another place I visited and added to my places-I-have-gone-and-now-have-an-opinion-about list. Gross.

The question of naming came up again. Ronnie said, Tenzin? No, I don't like that so much. Then my stepmother said, What are the kids at school going to call him? and my brother said, Ten. My father threw his hands up and said, I like Chaim, and I said, Dad, we talked about this, which we had, earlier in the day. I told him that I would not have anyone, including his grandfather, subjecting my child to even the merest hint of identity confusion. I said, What if Grandma had insisted on calling me Susan? And he paused and said, You're right, I would have told her that your name was Rebecca. But how is he going to get a job with a name like Tenzin?

You know, he said seriously, there is a group of women with names like Shanequa speaking publicly about how their names have kept them from succeeding in the workplace. They're all changing their names to Mary.

I told him that Tenzin was a perfectly respectable name, and part of a tradition at least twenty-five hundred years old.

Then I asked him how many jobs he thought Chaim would get, and we both burst into laughter.

September 26

The shower was yesterday. It blew me away. There were people from so many different parts of my life in one room, and for the first time I felt elation rather than dread at the thought of them all coming together. My East Coast family, the Yale mafia, the literary troupe, some Bay Area peeps who happened to be in the city, the buddies I got to keep after the big breakup, two rugged and beautiful idealists from the days I was running around raising money for nonprofits.

Even though I don't see many of them often, the people who came are definitely a part of my tribe, that ever-expanding crew held together by the resonance of a three-hour talk one night at a club about a relationship, or a series of conversations about a TV show we developed together, or a lunch about an essay that led to a discussion about marriage and kids and where the hell our lives were going. I've never felt happier to be surrounded by such a warm and loving bunch, or more certain I was in the exact right place at the right time.

And yet I kept thinking about the Langston Hughes line: What happens to a dream deferred? Does it dry up, like a raisin in the sun? What happens to all of these memories that dwell in the recesses of the mind like ghosts wandering the halls of some abandoned ruin? Where do these memories go, and what, if anything, do they ultimately mean? At the time, each of the encounters felt so meaningful, as if they were shaping the rest of my life, and yet they have all fallen away as mysteriously as they arose.

I can't help thinking of the shower that way, too. There was the idea of what we were doing, welcoming the baby and showering support and encouragement on the mom-to-be, and that is what we did. But the way we think of it, as a gathering that necessitates and facilitates the next gathering, and on and on until you've built a life, I didn't really feel that. It was more like the whole party was in a bubble flying over Manhattan, and when it was over, the bubble burst and then it was gone.

It reminded me of how I felt when I saw the vulture on the first day I found out I was pregnant. I feel as if the self I knew is fading away, and I have no idea who is coming to take her place.

September 29

Just back from a speaking engagement at Carnegie Mellon. Someone asked if I am experiencing pregnancy as the ultimate in Womanhood. It was an interesting question. I said that I feel more in touch with the animal qualities of the species, rather than the gendered ones. My sense of smell is heightened, I am ferociously protective of my developing offspring, my body is going through changes beyond my control in the service of species survival.

I told her that I really feel like an animal when I am hungry. In those moments, when I am on the hunt for my next meal, I feel out of control, led entirely by instinct. When I get to the food, I can barely observe basic etiquette. I want to tear at the meal, to wolf it down. And it's not all eco-friendly, either. I want big, thick, juicy steaks, and whole chickens. I want four scrambled eggs and six pieces of bacon. And then when I finish all that, I want a box of chocolate-covered donuts.

It's in the fact that instinct takes over, and the body is following intelligence all its own, that I find an inkling of an almost supernatural strength. I've always thought of myself as a pacifist. I painstakingly scoop up beetles and walk them outside. I tenderly coax house-trapped hummingbirds into my hand so that I can set them free without harm. But something else is activated in me now. I could kill someone standing in the way of my baby's fruition. It wouldn't even be that hard. The power to defend is that primal.

The women in the audience looked a little shocked, so I softened it a bit by talking about the other side. The way the pregnancy puts you smack in the middle of the huge mystery of life. The way you can't avoid the not-knowing, no matter how much the intellect tries to get a grip on the situation by taking tests and reading books. The way all you can do, really, is follow the cues you're getting from inside.

Ravenous, vulnerable, victorious. There is power in all of it.

I told her what I now tell lots of young women who look at me with the huge question mark on their face that I used to have: Being pregnant is the best. I highly recommend it.

I really do.

While your baby may soon slow up growing in length (he measures about 15.7 inches from crown to toe by now), he will continue to gain weight until he's born. . . . His lungs and digestive tract are nearly mature and he's probably been able to open and shut his eyes for a while now, so he can see inside you.

October 5

Talked for a long time last night with Glen. Seemingly out of nowhere I suggested we name the baby Jonah, or maybe David. He went through the roof. Um, hello? We're Buddhist, and more important than that, we made a decision. Please don't tell me your name ambivalence is stirred up.

But it's not ambivalence, it's guilt. I feel like I am letting down the clan. If the baby has a name that doesn't resonate with my family's biblical template, they may not bond with him. He's

going to need grandparents. Isn't it my responsibility as a mother
to make sure the seeds for these relationships are planted?

I also want him to relate to his roots, to know what it means to
be a part of this crazy tribe of people who mix love and arguing
like chocolate syrup and milk, who use Yiddish proverbs as terms
of endearment, and who manage to find fabulous YSL sandals in
the mountain of lame shoes at the Barneys warehouse sale.

Maybe guilt is the mechanism that holds families together. I
heard somewhere that human beings, in terms of the way we
organize ourselves, most resemble pack animals. As in wolves,
dogs, wildebeest. We want everyone in our pack to smell the
same. If they don't, we're not sure they're really one of us, and if
they're not one of us, how can we trust them?

Biblical name=Smelling the same
Smelling the same=Trust
Trust=Survival
———————————————
Biblical name=Survival

Sigh.

October 9

Sasha the birthing teacher came over today to teach us about
labor. She had lots of props: videos of women squatting their
babies out in Brazil, a miniature pelvis complete with slide-
through baby doll, a diagram of the ten most helpful positions a
labor partner can assume during a birth.

We learned about effacement and dilation and the three

stages of labor. We learned about breech births, posterior births, C-sections, and episiotomies. She had me hold a piece of ice in my hand to see how I managed the pain of ice burn. She encouraged me to talk about my fears, and to write down my hopes for the birth.

Two and a half hours into the four-hour class, Glen asked the quintessential question: "Where's the penis?" He said that everything thus far was about the vagina and the womb. Since the man was so involved in making the baby, there had to be an equally important role for him in the birth.

As Sarah sputtered about daddies being support people and being emotionally connected throughout the labor, I cracked up and looked at Glen with pride. It was such a classic Glen question, I just had to marvel at him.

We ended up having a long discussion of both the medical and natural childbirth models and the role they each have assigned to men. The medical model puts male doctors and a "masculine" institution in control, and the natural childbirth model relegates men to a relatively passive "support and behold" position.

Glen was interested in neither, and insisted there must be another option, something in between.

He mentioned the video of women squatting in Brazil, and asked Sarah if she had done any research in other cultures about the role of men in childbirth. I mentioned a tribe I read about in which men attach prosthetic babies to their stomachs while their partners are pregnant. During childbirth they beat themselves with dried leaves and branches to share the pain.

Glen raised his eyebrows. He wasn't sure about that, but he

liked the idea of looking more deeply into it. I made a mental note to add it to my already bulging list of potential article ideas.

All in all, the class was a good use of our time. By the time Sasha left, I was practically begging her to join my labor team. She's worked as a midwife all over the world and has assisted many, many births. She was smart and had excellent boundaries, which I always appreciate. But alas, she's traveling with her family in December, and can't make it.

But by then we may have discovered where the penis is in this whole process and won't need her!

October 12

Today a checker at the supermarket told me she is never having a baby. Because I am such a sucker for these random pregnancy conversations, I took the bait and asked why not. She can't stand the idea of dependency, she said. She never wants another human being to need her that much. The whole idea of it makes her sick. I asked her age. Twenty-three. I paused, considering my new role of crusader against maternal ambivalence everywhere. I tried to modulate my voice so I didn't sound like too much of a zealot, and told her she had plenty of time to change her mind. She looked at me as if I'd suggested that she cut off her right arm.

October 18

I met another doula today. She was warm and knowledgeable. She has been a doula for twenty years and is known as the best postpartum doula in the area because of the meals she cooks specifically to fortify breastfeeding moms. I liked her, but I am still not sure about opening up the intimacy of our family to a stranger. The more I think about another human being in our space, the more it feels, I don't know, awkward at best, intrusive at worst.

I told Dr. Lowen yesterday that I have officially decided to switch over to midwifery care for my delivery. She was sad to see me go and reminded me that she usually "lets" the mom have the second baby with a midwife, after they see how she does with the first. I left her office feeling guilty. Am I making a selfish decision that isn't best for the baby? Why are there so many goddamn decisions to make? And why do they all have such intense consequences? Is motherhood just another word for guilt?

Otherwise, the checkup was normal except that I am humongous. I've gained forty pounds so far and the nurse says I haven't even hit the heavy months yet. She said I am lucky because I'm carrying entirely on my stomach and not in my hips and butt.

Got home and puttered about. I cleaned out the refrigerator and all of the kitchen cabinets, and then moved on to reorganizing the hall closet. Spent an hour looking at beds online. Having a baby means that, in addition to a few other pieces of grown-up furniture, I must acquire a proper bed. It must have a headboard to lean against when nursing. It must be beautiful. It must have some kind of unseen storage element for baby blankets and baby clothes and all the rest of the baby stuff I am accumulating.

It must be sexy.

October 19

Tonight I drove myself to the drugstore for a nail clipper and another bottle of Tums.

Going out alone was eerie. I felt exposed in a way I've never experienced. Being a New Yorker, I am used to walking around at night. I know how to scan for danger without thinking about it. But I've never felt like I should be at home, behind closed doors, because the streets are unsafe. I definitely have never felt that I need to have a man by my side to protect me.

But that is exactly how I felt. It was brutal. I felt like my stomach made me a walking target, as if predators could smell my vulnerability. I had thoughts about being mugged, raped, or kicked in the stomach repeatedly. What an awful, awful way to hurt someone. When I think of all of the women and babies who have endured that kind of violence, my mind goes into spasm. I want to vomit.

Talked with Glen about it when I got home. He of course told me that I should not be driving around at night, alone, six and a half months pregnant. I was infuriated. I should be able to drive around any time I want and not have to worry about being bludgeoned to death. He agreed. You *should* be able to, he said, and hopefully one day you will. The real question is what are you going to do in the meantime?

Indeed.

October 22

Maybe it's that the rain hasn't stopped for three days, but today I am bored out of my mind. I am finally doing what everyone says I should have been doing for the last couple of months, resting, but it feels more like jail.

I have officially moved into the waiting phase of this pregnancy. Because even though I can go out and a part of me wants to go out, I really don't have the energy to go out. I would have to get showered and dressed, climb into the car, start it up, and will it down the freeway. No matter where I decide to go, I would have to acquiesce to being the center of attention. I'd have to pretend I was wearing a shirt with a big arrow pointing to my belly and "Ask me about my baby" emblazoned above it.

I am a lady-in-waiting. I am waiting for the big day, the big event, the arrival of the mystery. I know this is a sacred, spiritual time. I am reveling in the predawn of maternity. I am bonding with my baby. I am storing up energy for the upcoming marathon. I am taking care of myself by not exposing myself or the baby to violence, confusion, and chaos.

I know all of this, and I am grateful that I have the luxury to hole up and hide out. I don't have to do makeovers at the Macy's cosmetics counter, I don't have to harvest rice from sunrise to sunset, I don't have to sit in front of the computer fielding interoffice e-mails because I am worried that while I am on maternity leave someone will steal my job.

I know all of this, but still . . . All I can think about, besides being bored to death, is food. What can I eat next? In the last two hours I have had two bowls of chicken soup, three pieces of toast with chicken, two soy ice cream sandwiches, two huge glasses of organic lemonade, an apple, a pomegranate, and as I write this, I've got designs on a steak, a few pieces of sliced turkey, some brown rice, and an orange. Eat and wait. Eat and wait. Eat and wait. And watch movies. And answer e-mail. And write thank-you notes to the people who gave me gifts at my shower. And rub an infinite variety of oils on my bursting stomach to prevent stretch marks.

Glen says I am peripatetic and that he always knew this would be hard for me. "This" being the slowing down of my mind and body, the near cessation of my endless roam. I shake my head at him and think to myself that I understand that this is necessary for family life. I know I don't want to re-create my hypermobile childhood for this little baby.

But there is a secret part of me that thinks he might be right. Who are you kidding? the little voice says. You have a nomadic heart, do you not? You have learned that wherever you go that's where you are, but gosh, you sure like getting there and meeting yourself again.

Seven

TWO VERY POWERFUL and influential women were on television a few weeks ago, speaking triumphantly about the fact that they don't need men. I understand that. If you can financially provide for yourself, you are no longer dependent on another for economic support. I get it. But there are so many other kinds of support. When I think about trying to have this baby alone, without an intimate other to console me when I am worried and cook for me when I am so nauseated I can barely look at the kitchen, let alone stand in it, my head starts spinning. I understand the wisdom of having good friends to get these needs met, but really, I think we need partners in life.

I don't know if it's because I am a child of divorce, a Gen Xer accustomed to relating primarily though e-mail, or the daughter of a women's movement ambivalent about the institution of marriage, but until I met Glen, partnership was elusive. My relationships, while not lacking in intensity, lacked the magical togetherness quotient you find in healthily fused adults. I had never achieved the ineffable calm of couples that don't finish each other's sentences, not because they can't, but because they'd rather be quietly supportive of each other instead. I had never been half of a couple that checked in several times a day, no matter how mundane the conversation, to calibrate their movement as a unit from afar.

The most significant obstacle I faced to joining the club of the deeply, truly committed was my complete and utter ignorance of the importance of partner choice. I simply did not understand the necessity of intellectual compatibility and, even more important, *emotional reciprocity* in relationship. I now believe that there should come a time in every young woman's life when a more experienced loved one explains this absolute key point. It's not about marrying for love or money, it's about partnering for sanity, survivability, and the calculable probability that together the two of you will create something more gorgeous and powerful than you ever could alone.

There was also my religion to contend with: absolute autonomy. I would rather die than give up travel, sexual freedom, financial independence, and the cordoned-off secret section of my psyche where only I could go. I kid you not: When I met Glen, I thought I could have a baby with him and another with Ade in Africa, shuttling back and forth every six months. It wasn't until Glen reminded me that I almost died in Africa, and then gently suggested that my plan was completely unrealistic *in terms of maintaining intimacy,* that I realized I needed to get real and throw down the anchor.

I didn't have a visceral sense of what it might be like to merge with something or someone other than myself until I was thirty years old and listening to the Dalai Lama. He was talking about the myth of independence. If you are so independent, he asked, who grows your food? Who sews your clothes, builds your house, makes sure that water comes out of your showerhead? How were you even born? The fact is, he said, we have not done one single thing alone, without the help of a small army of others, and yet we walk around talking about the necessity and supremacy of independence. It's completely irrational.

For a brief moment I felt a softening of my self-perception, a relaxation of my ideas about where I stopped and other people began, a letting go into inseparability. I was not autonomous and never would be. What a relief! The Dalai Lama went on to say that no condition we find ourselves in is permanent. Rich people can become poor. Healthy people can become sick. Young people become old.

I flashed on this while watching the two women on television: the powerful and self-sufficient will become not so powerful and not so self-sufficient. These dynamic women for whom I have a tremendous amount of respect will both need someone at some point. I would wager that it would be more satisfying to them both if this someone did not have to be paid to show up.

I am not blaming feminism, because without parity and equality, partnership is just another word for exploitation. But I am suggesting we take another look at what we're thinking and saying in the name of "empowerment," and how that shapes our actual lives and impacts the people we love. As a mother, I worry about how it makes boys and men feel to hear they are not needed, and can be made obsolete by the presence of enough money and a few good girlfriends. I worry about how it makes them feel to hear that we don't care if they disappear from the face of the earth because we have enough frozen sperm to get us through the foreseeable future. And what about the millions of women who can't afford to not need men? Is empowerment impossible for them?

The more I learn about partnership, the more certain I am that the male partners of the women on television already put up with a tremendous amount of stress and strain just being the husbands of two very powerful, very visible women. Do you think they want to be more or less present, more or less intimate with their wives, after hearing that they aren't really necessary? I know how I would feel if the person I devoted my life to told millions of people he didn't need me.

Wrecked.

Because the fact is that we do need each other, and we are locked into this dance with the whole frickin' world whether we like it or not. This lack of separateness is awful and terrifying, amazing and exhilarating, and just plain true. It seems to me that men and women both need to come up to speed on this, instead of competing for the prize of who can do without whom for longer. There is power in partnership, otherwise the modern, government-sanctioned version of it, marriage, wouldn't be able to hold.

But I began this mini-manifesto simply because I have never felt as much dependence on another person, male or female, as I do now that I am pregnant. Granted, I do feel a tremendous power, a sort of Yes, I've got the fetus now, no one can stop me, but then when that necessarily subsides and I think about the thousands of decisions that are going to come up, the millions of moments where it will inevitably take two heads screwed on right to muddle through, I feel a tremendous need. To be a single mother, while I feel I could do it, at the moment seems an impossible task.

What I need is a partner: someone who will show up. And what I need to become is a partner: someone who will open the door. I have no idea if I can sustain it as long as I want, which is forever, but I've never felt so motivated to try.

October 24

Blessed be the editors, for they giveth work!

I spoke today with the editor of a high school English text-book I am writing an essay and teaching section for, and he put me on task. I have several subsections to write, answering questions like: What is the difference between an article and an essay? and What is my writing process like?

I decided to write the main essay for the textbook on hip-hop culture and what it was like before it became a global commodity. It's a personal piece about living in the Bronx in the eighties when it all began. And how, as a youth movement, hip-hop was about kids being free and expressive and having a good time. Most important, it was about kids from different cultures finding a common language.

Anyway. It's not like I don't have a whole other book to write, but it is nice to have a few short pieces to focus on. Otherwise,

I watch way too much TV. It's just so nice to lie about, clicking the remote. Right now I am in love with *Girlfriends* and *The King of Queens*. I'm convinced these shows are helping me bridge the chasm between single urban professional and suburban nuclear. My life at the moment is two parts *Girlfriends,* two parts *The King of Queens,* one part Discovery Channel.

Good news: I read on the Internet that mothers who eat a lot of chocolate when they are pregnant have happier babies.

November 4

The baby is super-awake today. I sense his awareness more than ever, that he's waking up and taking things in. I've started talking to him, out loud instead of just in my head. I tell him all of the things we're doing, like getting the car washed and driving to the chiropractor, buying laundry detergent and calling Grandpa on the phone. This morning I told him about Sonam and that she's going to be with us in the hospital. I told him not to be afraid because she has delivered hundreds of babies and she loves us.

It's all so exciting, but between interviewing doulas, training for the labor marathon, making sure I've got the right breast pump, and eating everything in sight, I'm totally exhausted. I get why people have their babies in the hospital. It's the planning, stupid! I feel like I'm making a Hollywood film with a two-person crew. If I were to have this baby at home, I would have to do all of what I am already doing, plus shop for plastic sheets and a fifty-foot hose for the water tank.

I'm finally convinced I've made the right decision. I just want to go to the hospital, have this baby, and then come home to a sane, stable environment. I know it sounds rough, but I have a hunch that giving birth is going to be hard enough. I don't also have to transform my apartment into a birthing center.

November 7

Since I haven't heard from my mother about the birthday tea since she brought it up two months ago, and since I've been feeling a bit sketchy about the whole thing anyway, I wrote her a note telling her that I don't feel comfortable moving forward with what I could only imagine wasn't really going to happen anyway, seeing as how my birthday is in ten days. I wrote that I am still having reverberations from all of the horrible things she said to me, and just don't feel safe. I apologized again for anything and everything I have done that has ever hurt her, and I thanked her for the offer, and I did all of the other nice things a daughter is supposed to do.

She wrote back: "Walk free, with my blessing."

November 8

I feel the inward turn today. I have no desire to do anything at all, other than eat, sleep, and dream. I have work to do and yet my brain does not cooperate. It wants only to lie here and contemplate the sky and the trees, to feel my baby move from side to side, to wonder about his face, his future.

November 10

Insomnia. My new bedtime is five a.m. I watch TV, read, scour the Internet for information about what the hell I am supposed to be doing and feeling this week. I worry. Can I really do this? What will become of me? Will I be trapped and miserable? I organize. I throw papers away, I order what I call "organizational principles" from the Container Store and make pretty, chronologically ordered file folders full of contracts, notes, articles, bills. I shred documents that I wouldn't want anyone else to see: medical records, first drafts, copies of tax returns.

I am up so much at night that it is starting to feel like day to me. Like I have collapsed the artificial line between day and night and I am living one long, seamless stream of life.

Another gift from Tenzin.

November 12

We nixed the postpartum-doula idea. We just don't want to have to deal with another person. I wish I could judge how incapacitated I will be. Some women I've talked to can't function for weeks and others get up after two days and do the grocery shopping. Where will I be on the spectrum? I have no idea. It all depends on the kind of birth I have.

In lieu of a doula, I figure I can get services lined up now so I won't worry about certain things. Like bottles of water. Fresh produce. Housecleaning.

Mr. T is moving around a lot today, kicking and elbowing me, his knees and tush sticking out from my belly. I started rubbing the parts that I can feel, massaging them and talking to him while I rubbed. He loved it.

November 19

We went to meet Sonam's backup doctor today, as required. When we arrived at her office in the Women's Center of the hospital, the small waiting room was packed with pregnant women about to pop. The doctors were running forty-five minutes to an hour late. There were no windows in the office, and the room was hot and stuffy.

To my left was a young woman ten days past her due date who kept shrieking, to no one in particular, It won't come out, it won't come out. She was accompanied by her mother, who looked stonily at the ground as her daughter screamed. At one point, this young woman asked another woman if her placenta was going to get stuck, and what she should do to make sure it comes out. The other woman very nicely told her not to worry, it would come out right after the baby.

There was a woman with a huge attitude talking on her cell phone to the father of her child. She told him that he needed to buy the baby some clothes or some formula since he hadn't done anything else for her the whole time she was pregnant. He said something and she said she didn't care about all that, all she knew was that he better buy something for this baby. Then she clicked her phone shut and went back to reading her magazine.

A young couple sat down next to us. They could have been in high school. The guy kept his arm around the girl the whole time we waited. She flipped through a magazine and they read it together, laughing sometimes, reading parts out loud to each other. Besides Glen, the guy was the only other man in a room full of hugely pregnant women.

About fifteen minutes before we were called in, a woman came in with her baby in a portable car seat. Turned out she was one of Sonam's patients. She said her birth went great, "You're gonna have a blast," which was the first time I had heard it put exactly like that. She also told me that it was all about the traveling car seat and that no, it wasn't too heavy.

I asked her how she was doing, and she said good. She tore a little bit, but it was all healed, and her energy was starting to come back. She said she was sweating all the time because her hormones were all over the place, and that nursing was harder than she thought it would be, but other than that she was loving being with her baby and it was all so much more normal and natural than she thought it would be.

Which was a relief.

Then the "It won't come out" woman asked her whether her placenta had come out on its own, or if she had to do something special to get it to come out, and the car-seat woman very patiently explained that no, you don't have to do anything special, it just comes out on its own after the baby. And the "It won't come out" woman nodded her head.

We were finally called in to meet with the doctor, who looked me over and said that for the most part everything looks fine and perfect and right on track, including the fact that I weigh 184 pounds. She said the low iron is still a problem. She's going to look into iron shots as a possibility but in the meantime told me to keep eating the beef, which I assured her I am, in copious amounts, thanks to Glen.

When she left the room, I started crying. It was just so intense in there. All those women. That young girl, probably developmentally disabled, not knowing what's going on. The tiny, airless office. Glen reminded me that we could be having the baby in the very nice, very airy hospital near our house. Which made me cry even harder.

November 24

I've started reading children's books. The Berenstain Bears, Richard Scarry, *Goodnight Moon.* The books take me back to purity, simplicity, ease. I remember why these books were my best friends when I was a little girl. Everything gets worked out, people love each other, the world is good.

I am reading these to counterbalance the e-mails that have been flying back and forth between me and my mother. I ask her to apologize for the dreaded afternoon and the statement she threatened to send to *Salon,* and to acknowledge the ways she has hurt me over the years with neglect, withholding, and the ambivalence she seems to have about my race, relative privilege, and birth itself.

She writes back that she has apologized enough and that children should forgive their parents and move on. She tells me that she and all of her friends think that because I have asked for this apology, I have lost my mind. I write her that asking people, even one's parents, to be accountable for their actions is the epitome of sanity, and that I am sorry that her friends, all of whom I know and love, don't have the courage to stand up to her.

When I write that if she can't apologize, I don't want contact because I feel she is too emotionally dangerous to me and my unborn son, she writes that she won't miss what we don't have and that to her our relationship has been inconsequential for years. She writes that she has been my mother for thirty years and is no longer interested in the job. Instead of signing "your mother" at the end of the letter, she signs her first name.

After that e-mail, I lie in bed trying to imagine some circumstance that could cause me to tell my child that I no longer want the job of being his mother. I think about Michael Jackson's mother, standing by his side in court as he responds to charges that he sexually molested children. I think about Scott Peterson's mother, who maintains that her son is a good boy even after he's been convicted of murdering his wife and child. Am I that awful, that I should no longer have a mother? Does telling my story the way I remember it make me a devil?

I try to imagine a circumstance that would lead me to tell my mother that I no longer want to be her daughter, that the job is just too draining, and I've found someone more suitable to take her place. When Glen walks in, I ask him to help me think, because, frankly, I am at a loss. I haven't even seen my baby and I feel I would die for him, kill for him if I had to. If I hurt him in some way, I imagine I would apologize to him over and over again until he could hear me, because that's what parents must do.

Glen sighs. It's not rational, honey, he says gently. An irrational person can find an endless number of reasons to justify ending a parent–child relationship, but a rational person knows that nothing can break that bond and it's madness to even try.

November 29

I am starting to think that giving the baby a Tibetan name isn't a betrayal of family as much as it is a sign of maturity.

Glen and I were flipping through a magazine, talking about how many people are stunted in their development, hovering in an adolescent state well into their fifties and sixties, even until death. He defined adolescence as being overly concerned with the acceptance of peers, and fearful of rejection or confrontation with the adult world.

Which made me think of how few people break away from the expectations of their parents to live their own, authentic lives. Guilt and fear keep so many of us ensnared. Who can stand the emotional blowback that comes from choosing a different path?

If guilt and fear keep us from acting on our own beliefs and aspirations, and not acting on our own beliefs and aspirations keeps us in a state of arrested development, there are bound to be some serious problems. If we aren't diligent in our efforts to mature, at some point cutting the cord of familial expectation, we become infantilized by it.

Sobering, but inescapable.

December 1

For research and recreation, I've been watching births on the Discovery Channel. It's amazing how many of these programs there are.

So far they fall into two categories:

The first is the normal birth. The mom lies calmly with her feet in the stirrups. She's completely epiduraled and everyone is just waiting, waiting, waiting until she's dilated. She looks content, and people come in and kiss her head and whisper in her ear. When it's showtime, the doctor comes in and peels back the sheet. He tells her to push. And push some more. Then we cut to commercial. Then we come back, and she's almost done. One more push, one more, there it is, yes! Congratulations, Samantha, you have a boy, a girl, a healthy baby. And everyone starts crying. If it's the home makeover show, this is when we cut to the almost-finished nursery, complete with gender-appropriate theme.

The second version is the complicated birth. In this segment, the mom does not look relaxed. She is on a gurney instead of a hospital bed. She looks panicked, in pain. She's practically crawling out of her skin. Doctors surround her and shout orders to nurses. Friends and family are remote. Then the decision to cut, to deliver by C-section. Mom is rushed to the OR, where a sheet is thrown over her legs so she can't see what's about to happen. Seconds later a bloody infant is held up, followed by applause, relief, exhaustion. Mom gets to rest her cheek on the baby for a few seconds and then, before we can wonder about the gash in her belly, we go to commercial.

Glen says I shouldn't watch, that it's like watching movies about plane crashes before taking a trip. But I am compelled.

He doesn't understand that I am measuring myself against the women I'm watching, trying to convince myself that giving birth is something I can actually do. When I watch the normal births, I say things to myself like, If she can do it, I can do it. I am tougher than she is. Oh, for God's sake, that's a piece of cake. When I watch the births with complications, I think: *Oh my God, I am never going to make it*.

I want to see a home birth, a natural birth. I want to see what it looks like with no anesthesia and no emergency C-section. What channel is that on?

December 2

It finally hit me that all of this nesting, this obsession with the right bed, the right stroller, the right house, the right amount of money, is about trying to control an absolutely uncontrollable situation.

It's about fear.

It is all in lieu of the actual work, which is to prepare to give birth the way I must prepare to die: alone. This morning at four forty-nine I realized that I alone am having this baby. Glen and the midwife will be in the room, but no one can come and do this for me, no one can make it not be hard, no one can make it not hurt. No one can bear the pain so that I don't have to.

The notion of waiting for someone else to bear your burdens, to save you—pregnancy is a lesson in the futility of all of that.

I feel relief, as if a huge burden has been lifted and I can let go of the superficial aspects of this pregnancy.

I feel like an adult.

December 4

Woke up this morning after the long, detailed meeting with Sonam, Glen, and Natasha, the masseuse and birth assistant I chose to be my doula, full of energy. I made a big breakfast, cleaned the kitchen, worked on the textbook piece, drove Glen to a doctor's appointment, went out to lunch, and kept going until five. I didn't realize I was in an altered state until later, when it dawned on me that the odd tightening across my big belly was my first set of contractions.

At six, I had a primal urge to be as close to Glen as possible, preferably with my face buried in his armpit, but not before eating an entire chicken, a loaf of bread, and two bottles of mineral water. I know it seems like I am exaggerating, and when I read this in a year I'll be like, Yeah right. I am not exaggerating. I really did eat that much. Tenzin, you have always been a healthy, strong, strapping boy.

Then at about two a.m., I had another very strong urge to complete all of my outstanding work. So I finished the textbook pieces and e-mailed them to the editor, and made a detailed list of the rest of the work to wrap up. I taped it on the wall next to all the other lists I've been compiling, and finally, after I read all of them over, tumbled into bed.

I dreamed that I went to the bathroom and looked down and there was my "bloody show." When I thought, *Oh my God, it's happening,* the baby slid out of me, right into the toilet.

December 6

Tonight I lay in bed thinking about the scarcity model versus the abundance model. For my whole life, I have operated as though there isn't enough love to go around, that love is something that must be stockpiled, hoarded, guarded for fear of losing a few precious drops. But lately, maybe because I've been contemplating what life would be like if I had, gasp, two or even three children, I have been thinking about how, while there may never be enough time or money, there will always be enough love.

What if everyone could let go of the fear and territoriality that comes from trying to control the love supply? What if everyone realized that love is about giving, not getting? What if everyone realized all of these things before it was too late?

What if it is true that when you believe in abundance, what you have multiplies magically?

December 13

Tomorrow is D-day and I don't feel any different than I have felt for the last couple of weeks: huge, heavy, and hungry. I thought I would have a premonition, or a sense of imminent arrival, but I just feel like, la-di-da, I am a pregnant woman waiting for my baby, who may or may not arrive at any moment.

In the meantime, I continue to prepare. I called the hospital today and pre-registered. I washed, folded, and put away all of the baby clothes, including six receiving blankets, twenty white onesies, three of the cutest little shirts with giraffes and monkeys on them, two little cotton hats, and a rainbow of the teeniest socks.

In packing the bag for the hospital I realized I haven't handled the nursing-bra situation, so Glen and I went to the mall and let the very nice saleswoman sell us a few. I even got one to wear at night while I sleep, which I cannot imagine doing, but the saleswoman was so certain I will need it that I couldn't leave it behind.

When we got home, I continued packing, and watched *The King of Queens* as I worked. Carrie finds out she is pregnant and is terrified they don't have enough money or maturity to have a baby. Doug gets really excited and vows to carry the financial burden by taking a second job. Carrie shops for baby furniture, and encounters a salesperson who convinces her that she absolutely needs, must have, a seven-hundred-dollar changing table with a safety lip. Doug takes a job driving a limo and gets as his first passenger the owner of CBS, who he thinks is the owner of CVS, the pharmacy. He passes out at the gynecologist's office because Carrie's no longer his sexy wife Carrie, she's more like the model of the impregnated uterus. They talk, convince each other it's going to be great. Doug buys a receiving blanket and comes home to find Carrie in the would-be baby's room, depressed. She lost the baby.

Even though I knew it was going to happen because I've seen the whole next two seasons and they don't have a baby, I was still hit pretty hard. Glen came in to find me on the edge of the bed, crying. Again.

If something happens to this baby I don't think I will make it. No, really. I don't.

December 14

No sign of *el muchacho*. Sonam came over to check me. When she walked in she said, You look like a mother today. And I grinned, because today I feel like a mother. I don't know when or how it happened, but I definitely have crossed over into mommyhood.

We talked about inducing. Whether we should, when we should, how we should. I don't want to rush him. I feel confident that he'll be right on time. On the other hand, I don't want to wait so long that it creates a problem. We came up with a plan: If he doesn't come by the twenty-second, we'll induce. He'll be a week late, which is still in the realm of healthy. In the meantime,

Sonam gave me a list of natural ways to induce, including sex, crying, and eating black licorice. I pinned it on the wall next to all the other lists I've made in the last eight months: Iron-rich Foods, Things For the Hospital, Five Best Things Your Partner Can Tell You When You're Pregnant.

Sonam also said that I must get more sleep. It's hard, though, because the baby wakes up at night and I'm right there with him. His body isn't moving, but I can feel his mind. He's waiting, listening, being.

December 16

I assembled the co-sleeper today. And then I stared at it for an hour, unable to imagine what it will feel like to have a real, live baby lying next to me at night.

I can see him now, not the details, but the blur of his face. And we've been talking to each other. Ready? Ready. Ready? Ready.

Today I caught myself singing to him. At first it was "Michael, Row Your Boat Ashore," and then it was both of the Color War alma maters that I can remember from summer camp, and then, I am embarrassed to even write this: "Kumbaya." But I sang that one only because I couldn't think of any other songs besides "You Are the Sunshine of My Life," "You've Got a Friend," "Isn't She Lovely," and "Let's Stay Together."

How is it possible that I don't know any lullabies? My father's friend George gave me ten CDs of lullabies from all over the world. Obviously, every other woman on the planet has lullabies welling up naturally from the depths of her soul. Why don't I have a whole repertoire, in multiple languages? When I asked

Glen he said, I don't recall the baby asking you to sing him a medley of lullabies from around the world.

Which is true, and made me laugh.

People have been calling every day now that I am past the due date. Is he here? How are you doing? Sweet to feel them in the space with me: waiting, waiting, waiting.

Eight

I MET GLEN at a meditation retreat. I was tearing through a plate of organic greens and tofu lasagna in the dining room of the retreat center when I turned my head slightly and caught sight of him. He was three empty chairs away, and wore the burgundy robes of a Buddhist tradition I didn't recognize. He had a full beard, large hands, and soft brown eyes.

Ordinarily I would have turned away, but because we were up in the mountains with only each other and sixty or so others for company, I did not. I smiled when our eyes met and paused, taking him in. He too was quiet, not rushing to fill the space. Then in the least intrusive but most penetrating voice I've ever heard, he said hello. I gave a slight bow. Hello. And then we didn't speak for the rest of the meal.

I saw him next the following morning, at the early teaching. I was groggy from lack of sleep, but I noticed Glen right away when I walked into the meditation hall. He was sitting off to the side, looking at and seemingly through the entire group of assembled students. He was purposefully threading a thick, rose-colored *mala* through his fingers. He was so still he was practically invisible.

That morning, I listened respectfully to the teaching, but really I was already attuned to Glen, and found myself glancing over at him several times during the two-hour session. When it was finally his turn to teach, I felt a curious mixture of excitement and readiness. This is a cliché, but when he began to speak, I really did feel as though he was speaking only to me. When he sang a *doha,* an ancient song calling all beings to enlightenment, I wept.

A year later we sat in a Japanese restaurant. We had not been out of contact for more than a day since the afternoon in the dining room. As is customary in the teacher–student relationship in the Vajrayana tradition, Glen had committed himself to transmitting to me some of the most esoteric of Buddhist teachings, and I had committed to deepening my devotion to him in order to receive them. As is customary in the romantic tradition of modernity, as my lover Glen had committed himself to making me happy and I had almost committed to letting him.

I was open but a bit unsure. I had heard horrible stories about teachers and students who became involved. There were messy, public lawsuits, and whole websites devoted to documenting incidents of "sexual misconduct." Family members expressed concern. I listened, but ultimately had to acknowledge that in the midst of so much doubt, no one could deny that I was happier than I had ever been. In one year, I had healed relationships that had been broken for decades, and jettisoned relationships that had no possibility of coming around. My work was more satisfying. I fired my therapist. I smiled more in one day after meeting Glen than I had in a whole year before.

And he wanted to have a baby.

I had told him shortly after our meeting just like I had told everybody else: *I want to have a baby*. But unlike everyone else, he responded decisively. Of course you want to have a baby, he said, and you should. There are things you learn when you have a baby that you cannot learn any other way. You find out what life is about when you carry another human being in your womb. You find out what really matters when you straddle life and death to push your child through the birth canal.

I told him about my list of potential daddy donors, about Ade. I told him about the abortion I had when I was fourteen and my fear that I would not be able to conceive. I told him about Solomon. We talked about the years I had spent running from potential mates and devoting my life to people completely unsuited.

We talked for hours every day, and it was as if the years slid off me with each conversation. Self-concepts were reevaluated. The constant loop of self-deprecation that had been running in my head for decades grew less and less audible. When Glen wondered why I didn't listen more attentively to my ten-year longing, I asked myself the same question. What would it mean for me to have a baby? What would the experience reveal? Why did I crave it so profoundly? After several months, I began to wake up in the morning believing that having a child was not only possible, but necessary.

One day in my icebox of a writing studio by the sea, I told

Glen of a dream I had been having for several years. There was a little boy, sleeping in a cave, and there was an angry woman, stabbing at my heart. The boy was waiting patiently for me to come, and the woman was trying to prevent me from getting there.

Glen stood in front of a huge panel of my printed pages thumbtacked to the wall in a neat row of white rectangles, nodding as I described the colors in the dream, the sound of the knife slicing through the air. When he finally did say something, he didn't so much decipher the dream as join me in the labyrinth of it.

He wondered if my happiness was dangling in the space between the boy and the woman trying to keep me from him. Who was she and how could I get past her? Who was he? On reflection, it occurred to me that this boy curled up in the invisible space around my body could be *my* boy. He slept peacefully, patiently, as if he knew for certain that I would come. As if he knew that I would slay the dragon and vanquish the enemy, that the fight would end and we, he and I, would win.

This little boy knew what I was only just beginning to suspect. That with Glen I was healing something that had been broken for a very long time: my ability to trust, my right to dream. I was repairing my broken faith, but it was still far from restored. Which is why I laughed nervously into my tempura udon when Glen told me that I had found the father of my child and could stop looking.

I was thirty-three. I had been considering having a baby for more than ten years. I had finally met someone who was willing and able to give me the partnership I craved, and I was scared to death. Scared of closing an unseen, imaginary door by walking through the very real, open one in front of me. Terrified of following a vision that had beckoned for more than a decade.

Could I even take care of a child? When I looked back, there were so many broken relationships, stories that started out shiny and happy just like this one. But now there would be a vulnerable child in the balance.

As if reading my mind, Glen suggested that the healing would come through my not doing to my child what was done to me. Not succumbing to divorce. Not forcing my child to adapt to wildly divergent circumstances to suit my lifestyle. Not arguing. Not making him hold the unresolved issues of the generations that preceded him. Not forcing him to choose which parent to believe, to trust, to become.

If I could do this on behalf of my actual child and the neglected child inside of myself, the demon would have no choice but to put down her knife. My child would awaken and live. I would know how to protect myself. The cutter, the mutilator, would not be allowed inside.

I knew Glen was right, but I was also frightened of making a conscious decision, a reasoned choice. I had lived my life tumbling headlong into scenarios, captivated by ideas like fate and romantic love. What did it mean to decide, after extensive evaluation and discussion, to move forward together, instead of waking up one morning to realize that yet another boundary had been crossed and I was now deeper into a relationship that I really did not fully understand?

I loved Glen deeply. But because I was with him engaged in the project of giving up drama forever, our relationship was disturbingly stable, calm, rational. When I told my father about Glen, he said that our relationship sounded good but that something was missing. We were walking arm in arm around the lake in Central Park. It's clear that you love this person, he said, stopping by one of the benches. But Rebecca, tell me, are you in love with him?

At the time, I brushed it off. In love? I've been in love, and where has that gotten me? We laughed, but my mind seized on the question as we navigated the throngs on Fifth Avenue. I've met a man who has brought me more happiness than I imagined possible, who has offered to give me the one experience I've craved my whole life, who has stood by my side through depths of despair so profound I was afraid to mention them for fear of shattering your faith in yourself as a parent, and you ask if I am in love with him?

Loving, being in love. The whole idea of a difference between the two suddenly struck me as preposterous. And yet, if I wasn't intoxicated, swept off my feet, was I settling? Was I like other women who had reached a certain age—in my case, thirty-three—and found themselves in need of a certain sperm donor daddy type? Was Glen just a prudent and convenient choice?

This was the voice of the woman with the machete. Always slashing to bits whatever piece of happiness I managed to find. Was she my mother? This was the voice of my father's pervasive ambivalence, transmitted from one generation to the next through innocent conversations like the one in the park.

I slurped my noodles.

I put the woman's own knife to her neck and bade her farewell.

I leapt with certainty into the void.

Nine months later, I was pregnant.

LIKE ALL COUPLES, Glen and I have gone over that first hello a thousand times. We've marveled at how, of all the people present, we ended up next to each other, with empty seats and not obscuring human bodies in between. We've excavated the back story: Glen hadn't planned to go to lunch at all that day, but changed his mind and turned into the dining room instead. I hadn't planned to go to the retreat at all, but changed my mind and drove myself the seventy-five miles from the city.

At the retreat, though joined by a common interest in Buddhism, we were in distinctly different camps. I was with a group of women practitioners who visited the retreat center regularly and had for many years. He had never been on the property and was there because his students, most of whom were men, had implored the head teachers to invite him. With a word, we breached the space between territories and created a whole new world, separate and distinct from both.

Are we reading too much into it? Perhaps. But I have yet to meet a couple that didn't feel the echoes of destiny, fate, angels, or, as Buddhists call it, karma. Buddhists don't believe in a god up in heaven moving people around like chess pieces across the universe. But we do believe in cause and effect: that each moment is very much the result of all the moments that came before.

In one cosmic moment, we stepped into the stream of our son's potential for being. We decided to say hello, and the rest, as they say, is history.

Or Tenzin's story.

baby boy who is undeniably the most precious being I have ever seen.

I honestly don't know if I can bear it.

His name is Tenzin Walker.

Suffice it to say, all is not peaches and cream. Tenzin is in the neonatal intensive care unit, but I am too exhausted to write the entire saga, so it will have to wait until tomorrow.

December 23

The Entire Saga:

Yesterday at five o'clock I was so hungry I felt I could eat the headboard off my new bed. Glen brought me what I craved: quick, greasy take-out that I ate with abandon. A huge hamburger with onions, bacon, and cheddar cheese, a Greek salad, and two orders of french fries disappeared within minutes.

At seven, I was checking e-mail and noticed the vivid purple and red streaks of the sunset outside my window. I felt relieved that I had cleared all the writing assignments from my desktop. I went to the bathroom and saw a little blood, not a clot, but enough to think that something might be happening. I called Glen and then Sonam, who asked if there was a lot of fluid. I said no and she said it may be starting, but maybe not. She told me to breathe, stay calm, and keep in touch.

I made it to the bed before the first contraction hit. It was like the contractions I had been having except this one extended beyond my belly deep into my pelvis. It was slightly orgasmic, and I thought that if this was it I couldn't imagine why anyone would want to have an epidural. Then the contractions started coming every ten minutes or so, with growing intensity. After forty-five minutes, I could no longer sit still. I asked Glen if this was it, was it happening, and he said, Could be, but let's just stay calm and wait and see.

He got a little pad out and started taking notes, and I got really upset. Of course, I was writing cryptic messages to myself in my tiny blue notebook, but him doing the same thing made me feel like an animal under observation. I got pissy and he said I was trying to control his experience. I had a flash of depression: Were we really going to have an argument as I was going into labor?

No.

Once he put the notebook away, labor took off like a rocket and I couldn't hold on to any thoughts at all. The contractions started coming faster. There was a two- or three-minute break between them, but after the first minute, I dreaded the coming of the next one and began to clench in anticipation.

I called Sonam again and told her how fast they were coming. She said it sounded like I was in labor and she was going to pack her bag and come over. The pain started to get super-intense. I had a strong urge to take off all my clothes and lie in the bed with Glen until it was all over, but the only way I could survive the contractions was to keep getting up and sitting down. Then one of them hit and hurt so much that I fell to my knees. I spent the next two hours going from the floor of the bathroom to the toilet.

Sonam arrived and found me on all fours on the bathroom floor. She checked me and said that I was completely effaced and already a few centimeters dilated. She said we should get ready to go to the hospital. I didn't think I could get to the front door, let alone the hospital, and I think I screamed that out, along with some other unsavory epithets.

Glen swung into high gear, getting the food bags and my hospital bag and my coat and blankets and pillows covered with garbage bags in case my water broke in the car. I kept calling for him and he kept coming back to the bathroom every few minutes to tell me he was getting everything ready and that now was the time to execute our plan, not rethink it. Which would have made more sense to me if I could have executed getting off the bathroom floor.

From somewhere far, far away, I think the living room, I heard Sonam call Natasha and tell her that we would be at the hospital within the hour and she should go over and start setting up the birthing pool. That sounded so reasonable, but it also sounded like Sonam and Glen were both completely out of touch with reality. In between contractions, I told them so in a conversation I had with them in my mind. In our little imaginary chat, I told them that there was no way I could leave the bathroom floor, and we should prepare to have the baby in the bathtub. I had plenty of towels and there was a toilet and a shower and they were both there and, well, what more could we possibly need?

But then Glen and Sonam were helping me up and leading me to the car, and I was grabbing all kinds of random things like scarves and little bottles of massage oil and my favorite socks with the anti-skid patches on the bottom and several notebooks until Glen cut through it all and said, Rebecca, we have to go right now. And I thought, *Okay, got it. I can't back out of this, I can't procrastinate, I've got to just get with the program and get my ass in the car.* Then we were in the car and speeding along in the dark and I literally thought I was going to die. The contractions were coming in waves and the pain was so intense and unbearable I couldn't do anything but scream and freak out and lose my mind when they hit.

Which is what I was doing when we drove up to the emergency room and a security guard offered to get me a wheelchair. I said no, thanks, and then he asked again, directing his question to Glen and I almost tore his head off. I don't want a wheelchair, I screamed. Just open the door and tell me where to go.

I don't remember being in the elevator but I do remember Natasha coming down and getting all of our bags and I remember getting to the room and throwing myself onto the futon. After a few minutes, the contractions forced me to my hands and knees and I started crawling around screaming that I couldn't believe all human beings came here this way and that every single mother had to go through this.

Sonam and Natasha were calm and trying to help, but it was not at all like I thought it would be, with soft lights and my aromatherapy atomizer spritzing lavender-scented negative ions into the room and Natasha rubbing my back and Glen whispering in my ear and Sonam directing nurses and giving me visualizations. It was chaos and mayhem, and there was no room in the experience for anyone but me. I asked Natasha to rub my feet and arms and legs, and she tried for about forty seconds before I ran to the toilet and then decided that what I wanted—no, *desperately needed*—was to take a shower.

Glen turned the water on and stood with me while I gripped the safety rail, lay my head on the plastic wall, and wailed that I didn't think I could make it. Then I got into the birthing pool, the thing I thought would be my salvation, and it was, for about ten minutes. Then it got too hot and I couldn't move around enough so I had to get up and go back to the bathroom.

By this point it must have been one or two in the morning and we had been going since eight. I got up on the bed and hit the toilet a few more times and then Sonam checked me and said I was about four centimeters and we needed to get to eight, and that's when I realized there was no way I could do it. I was exhausted and it hurt so fucking much and I just couldn't believe that I had so much more to endure. I looked at Natasha, Sonam, and Glen standing respectfully at the periphery of my experience, in it with me, but only as far as they could be. Then I said, really loud, *I want an epidural.*

The three of them looked at each other, not sure what to do. Looking into their blank faces, I reminded them that I asked them to get me an epidural if I wanted it. They started to deliberate, and then to try and talk me out of it. At which point I began to plead for the epidural. Please, you guys, don't make me beg. Just get me the epidural. I have got to have the epidural. Please go get me the epidural.

The moment Sonam went to get the anesthesiologist, I started to feel better. It still hurt like bloody hell, but I knew it was going to end and that gave me a moment's respite from the horrifying thought that I was going to be in this god-awful pain forever. The sun started to come up and the room got very still, punctuated by me screaming at anyone who entered the room: Are you the anesthesiologist? Get the anesthesiologist. When is the anesthesiologist coming? Where is the anesthesiologist?

I have never been as happy to see another human being as I

was when the anesthesiologist walked over to my bed and told me to sit up so that she could insert the epidural. I was almost weeping with gratitude. She introduced herself and told me what to expect and I felt a stick and some jostling at the base of my spine and heard some tape being pulled from a tape dispenser. The nurses were talking to each other but I started to lose track of what they were saying, and slowly, slowly the pain began to lessen until I was relaxing in an extremely pleasant haze, and Glen was rubbing my forehead and telling me to take a break and get some rest.

That was lovely.

I floated in and out of consciousness for a while, and everyone took a breather because I was calm and not crawling around like a madwoman. Glen called my father and left messages for a few friends. Sonam got some juice. Natasha rubbed my feet and fluffed my pillows. The nurse had me breathe some extra oxygen and told me I was doing great. Then, just as I was really getting into it, and thinking I was finally going to be able to get some sleep, Sonam checked me and said that I was fully dilated and it was time to push. She said it might be hard to feel the contractions because of the epidural, but that I was going to have to really focus and try my best.

Even though I didn't want to go back to work, I was game to push because I thought that meant I was almost done. After what I had just gone through, how hard could pushing be? I got up on my elbows and grabbed Glen's hand and started giving it my all, bearing down and grunting and straining and making hideous faces, none of which had any effect whatsoever. I couldn't feel anything below my waist. The baby wasn't moving, but Sonam did see that he was posterior, turned around, which was going to make everything even harder.

Right around this time, when Sonam was telling me that a shot of Pitocin would intensify the contractions and make pushing easier, the nurse started getting adamant about the oxygen. The numbers coming out of her machine were not good, and suggested the baby was going into distress. His heart rate was down, which meant he wasn't getting enough oxygen. I could tell that she was a little concerned, but trying to make it sound totally normal so I wouldn't fall apart. This was not effective. I believe I started to say "What is wrong with the baby?" over and over again and when they told me, I tried to take in the oxygen, but the mask was so awkward and uncomfortable that it was hard for me to push, worry, and breathe at the same time. The Pitocin started to kick in and so did the pain. I pushed and pushed until I couldn't stand it anymore and then Sonam went to find the anesthesiologist to top off my epidural.

At that point, time began to be a major issue. The nurse's machine was beeping and she kept putting the oxygen over my face and doctors started coming into the room to see what was going on and provide backup. I was making a little headway with the pushing, but not much. The baby would come out a little and then go back. He did that several times, until I was completely exhausted and didn't think I could do any more. That was when I started saying, Just cut me open and get the baby.

Then he made it out a little farther, but got caught under my pelvic bone on the right side. Which hurt like hell, in addition to all the other hurting like hell going on. Then he and I did the

"Okay, let's get you out from under my pubic bone" dance for what seemed like an eternity. I was pushing so hard I thought the sides of my head were going to burst open. I was pushing so hard I thought I was going to knock myself unconscious. I was pushing so hard and I still couldn't feel the baby coming out.

The room was filling up with people but I couldn't focus on who they might be or why they were there. Sonam's backup doctor came in completely covered in OR blues and stood very close to me, speaking directly into my ear. She said, The baby is in distress. If you can't get the baby out in the next few pushes, we are going to have to do a C-section. Do you understand what I am saying? I looked at Glen and he was stable and calm, and then I heard Sonam tell the doctor that she knew I could do it. She is definitely going to get this baby out, she said.

The only thing I could think to do was get on my hands and knees and try to get him out that way. Sonam was yelling, Push your baby out, Rebecca. Bring your baby into the world, Rebecca. Come on, push. I could feel all the people in the room watching, suspended in the moment. I had a flash that I should feel embarrassed about being naked on my hands and knees in front of a room full of strangers, but honestly, I couldn't have cared less. Really. It was more like, I hope they understand that they are experiencing a goddamn miracle right now. It doesn't get more real than this.

Then time opened up, the seconds expanded into a dozen dimensions, and everybody in the room fell into it. At the exact moment I thought I was going to collapse and be wheeled into the OR and cut open, I felt the baby's head pop free and Sonam said, That's it, one more big push, one more, come on. And I pushed and then he was slithering out of my body and everyone in the room broke into applause and I started crying and fell back onto the bed.

People were making all kinds of oohing sounds and Sonam said, You did it! You had a healthy vaginal birth! Then she asked if Glen wanted to cut the umbilical cord. Glen said yes and took the scissors and did a blessing over the baby in Tibetan. With one snip, me and my boy went from one to two. Sonam placed him on my chest and the two of us lay there together, exhausted.

He was breathing heavily and looking around with calm curiosity. I couldn't see him so much as feel him, his slippery, smooth torso and floppy limbs. And his mind, I felt his perfectly open and clear mind. He was so present, so unencumbered by ideas about what he was seeing that I felt I was holding a being from another planet.

Then they took him away from me and I started to hear doctors mumbling about meconium and they asked Glen to go with them to the NICU and then I was just lying there, with a gaping hole in my belly and no baby in my arms.

When I arrived at the NICU, the nurses brought me over to Tenzin. I almost broke down. He was completely naked, strapped under an oxygen tent with tubes and monitor leads coming out of his arms and legs. He looked cold, even though there was a warmer over him. The right side of his face was bruised, and skin was peeling off all over his body. His breathing was so labored that his chest and neck lifted off the table each time he took a breath. I couldn't touch him because he couldn't come out of the tent, but I got close to the plastic cover and told him that Mommy was right there and he didn't have to worry and he'd be better soon.

He didn't move. I thought I was going to pass out. The word "agony" doesn't begin to capture what I felt.

Because the neonatologist wasn't there yet, the only thing I could do was talk to the nurse assigned to him and try to forge a bond. I hoped that my love and concern would be transmitted through her to the baby. Then I went to my little hospital room filled with unopened bags of stuff I thought was so essential to labor and passed out.

Four or five hours later, one of the neonatologists, Dr. Morales, came into our room. She said that Tenzin has meconium, the first waste product of the baby, in his lungs and that is making it hard for him to breathe in enough oxygen. He's getting oxygen now under the tent, and they've started him on a round of antibiotics to ward off infection. She said he is very vigorous, and has a very strong cry, which is a good sign. She said that babies with meconium are usually in the hospital for a week to ten days. She said we just have to watch him and hope the meconium cycles through and that he will be able to breathe on his own soon.

December 24

There are three neonatologists here who rotate. We met the second today. Turns out he is the father of an old college class-mate, which is vaguely comforting.

Anyway. Dr. Thompson came into my room and we had a long talk. He thinks Tenzin had meconium in his lungs before he was even born, and that once he began to breathe, it corrupted the lung tissue. He said there was no meconium in the amniotic fluid so they didn't realize that he needed to be intubated at birth. I wanted to say no, it wasn't that there wasn't meconium in the fluid. There was no fluid. My water didn't break at all, probably because Tenzin was further past term than any of us thought and should have been induced.

But I didn't say that and instead just tried to listen to him without panicking. He described the meconium as tarlike and extremely noxious. If Tenzin breathed it in for several minutes, which he must have because he was on me for at least that long, there may be some lung damage. He says it is unlikely, and usually babies with meconium aspiration syndrome (MAS) go home after their time in the NICU breathing normally and have no long-term effects. He said the X ray shows that the right side is more "involved" than the left, which makes sense because that was the side that was hurting so much during labor, the side that got hooked under my pelvic bone.

I am able to process what the doctors tell me about Tenzin, but I must be in shock because that is all I can do. I can't believe how hard the labor was and how unprepared I was for it after all of that preparation. I can't believe he's in the NICU. I can't believe I am not nursing my baby right now, bathed in the idyllic glow of postpartum. Instead, I feel like I've been in a car accident.

I went online and put in "in utero meconium aspiration." The first listing that came up was "in utero meconium aspiration: an unpreventable cause of neonatal death."

THERE WILL BE no neonatal death on my watch.

Janet the breastfeeding consultant brought me a big yellow breast pump today. Even though I've gone over breastfeeding on the antidepressant a dozen times with Marie, Dr. Lowen, Sonam, and anyone else who would listen, I had to get another opinion from Janet, who referred to a book she carries in her pocket that says that the benefits outweigh the risk. I revved up the pump and got to work. Just a little colostrum, but it was enough to put in a bottle and take over to the NICU to store in the fridge.

Storing food for the babe. Check.

December 25

Babies are flying through the NICU today. Every couple of hours there is a new "Jesus" or "Christopher" from the mostly Catholic moms. A volunteer group knits hats for the newborns, and so the baby Jesuses are lying in their plastic bassinets with tiny green and red caps on. Christmas isn't my thing, so I picked a nice beige one for Tenzin when his nurse, Rose, offered. Rose is from the Philippines and is very auntie-like. She talks to Tenzin in a singsongy voice, very loud, which seems to get his attention, and assures me he's going to be fine when I stare at him with longing and worry.

Tonight was better than last night, primarily because they've taken the oxygen tent away and given him a cannula that threads around his head, so at least he's not like the boy in the bubble. I can touch his forehead and rub my nose against his cheek. His breathing is still extremely labored, but so far everyone tells me he's quite vigorous for a baby as sick as he is, a good sign.

I was supposed to go home today, but Sonam managed to get me an extension, and then the hospital offered me a room for after that. They have a rooming-in policy for moms with sick babies. I can have a room close to the NICU as long as they don't need it for an incoming mom. I feel such gratitude for this humane policy, and wonder if the fancy, more expensive hospital has a similar policy. I don't know what I would do if I had to leave him every day. I don't think I could survive it.

December 26

It's two a.m. and I think I am having a nervous break-down. I paged Natasha 911, and when she called I told her every-thing and she said it's all normal. Most women crash around day three postpartum. It's when all the feel-good hormones you've been carting around with the baby inside suddenly plummet, never to be seen or heard from again. I cannot wake Glen up again with another string of woes, but really, I feel unfit to be a mother, and that I failed at giving birth. If I hadn't been so pigheaded about natural childbirth, I might have known that he was late and had him induced, and then we might not be going through this. I refuse to beat myself up, and then I start swinging.

If all that wasn't enough, I hurt in so many inconvenient places it is ridiculous. I can't walk a step without feeling like my uterus is going to fall on the floor, and my lower back, where the epidural went in, is *killing* me. I could take a Vicodin to take the edge off, but the pain doesn't seem intense enough to justify pass-ing a narcotic on to the baby. Sonam's backup midwife checked me this morning and reminded me that this is the kind of back pain that makes epidurals problematic. I didn't say anything, but I thought I would have to be damn near paralyzed to think twice about having another epidural. As far as I am concerned, that needle saved my life.

I am completely sick of dealing with blood and urine and shit and milk. It's like my whole body has been reduced to a quintet of oozing sores. And where is my baby? Where is my baby? Where is my baby?

. . .

I COULDN'T TAKE IT. I had to be near him, so I went over to the NICU and watched him sleep. His vulnerability is heartbreaking. I don't understand how human beings have survived these feelings for millions of years. How mothers have survived losing their sons to war, their daughters to marriage and relocation, and their children to disease and famine.

When I was in my twenties, my mother told me that she had to decide to love me, that she could have gone either way and she *chose* to love me. At the time, her words seemed strange, but I had no reference point so I just nodded and felt grateful that she'd made the choice that didn't leave me motherless. Seeing Tenzin's vulnerability makes me shake my head in wonder at her disclosure. There is no choice involved in my love for Tenzin, and if there were some secret place where I wondered, and there isn't, I would never tell him about it.

What I will tell Tenzin one day is that his need for me and my love for him are by far the most powerful human truths I have ever known. I would give my life for his in a heartbeat, and in some ways I think that is what is happening. Giving birth *was* like dying and being reborn. I went into labor one person, and came out two. I went into labor with a singular consciousness, and came out with a consciousness that transcended my own. I understand now the Tantric teachings on giving birth to your enlightened mind, and why the feminine is exalted in those teachings. Women can literally give birth and, through this process, birth an expanded understanding, a more enlightened, transpersonal view.

I thought there would be loss and mourning involved in the abandonment of my preoccupation with myself, but so far, even with the unbelievable pain and complications, it is all gain. I feel lighter, clearer about what needs to be done, and what my role is in the whole big, astonishing universe. Tenzin is my son and I am his mother. Is there anything else?

December 27

I am feverish today, sweating and shivering. My breastfeeding book says it could be milk fever, which makes sense because my breasts are like giant gourds. Really. They are astoundingly, almost obscenely engorged, painful to touch, and just, I don't know, so intense. When I walk, it's like I am a pair of breasts walking with a body attached. They lead when we enter a room, demanding acknowledgment and respect from all who come near.

Did I mention that they hurt?

I started pumping a couple of days ago, when Janet told me to store the colostrum, but today the floodgates have opened. I am now pumping every couple of hours, and filling bottles and bottles of milk. If I don't pump, I leak until I am drenched. Every time I walk over to the NICU to put another bottle in the fridge, one of the nurses says, Another one?

So here I am, scribbling this as I sit on the edge of the bed with my breasts stuck into mechanized suction cups strapped to my body with an elastic pumping bra. I feel like a cow, but every time I fill up another bottle I have a brief moment of ecstasy. My body is producing food for my baby. It doesn't get much better than that. Well, maybe it does. I'd rather be nursing. That would make a great bumper sticker to stick on this pump.

I'd rather be nursing. Yeah.

December 28

Not good. Tenzin is not improving and we have moved on to check for other possible diagnoses. Roth ordered a cardiac echo, which will check to make sure the valves in his heart are working properly and that the one that is supposed to have closed by now has done so.

That was sobering news. I settled in a little more after hearing that. When I was thinking we'd be going home in a week, I was more transient, mentally, but now it could be weeks.

I've moved into a new room because Labor and Delivery filled up and they needed my old one. This room is pretty rustic and has a mysterious leak in the floor. Getting out of bed this morning, I stepped in a huge puddle. After I told the nurse, a very nice man came to mop the water up, but within fifteen minutes the water was back. Then the engineer came up and said he couldn't figure out where the water was coming from. I told him I don't really care about the water, I just want to be close to my baby.

I unpacked the rest of my stuff here in the new room: food and robes and slippers and shirts and salves and medicines and baby clothes I thought Tenzin would be wearing by now. I burst into tears, and then I briefly considered going online. Friends and family have been calling and writing, but I don't have the energy to give them the details. I need to keep my mind clear and focused on being there for the baby.

December 29

I am starting to feel closer to the nurses, especially Gemma and Rose, and I've struck up a friendship with another mom. I don't know her name, but her baby was born two months premature the day before Tenzin. This is her fourth child, and she's already up and back to work. She comes in the evenings to give the baby a bottle, sometimes with her husband. When she arrives, I give her whatever update I can. Like if her little girl was peaceful or ate a lot. And she asks if Tenzin is getting better. Did he gain weight? Have they lowered the oxygen? Then we sit there, not more than five feet between us, staring at our babies and willing them to be okay.

Gemma told me today that she was born in the Philippines and then went to work as a nurse in Dubai, where she met her Surinamese husband. They have two kids, a boy and a girl. The boy had meconium and is now totally fine, with no residual problems. She showed me a picture of him as proof. He's beautiful. Her little girl is three months old. She said she's jealous of all my milk (One of the nurses joked that they need a whole fridge just for Mommy Walker!) because she is pumping at work and not getting much, only three or four ounces. I can get out three ounces in three minutes.

We talked about how difficult it is to work full-time and raise two kids. She thought America would be different, but she has to work so much to pay for her mortgage and for the kids' schools.

She said the quality of life was much better in Dubai (!). It is interesting to hear about the American Dream through the prism of her life. So far, I think she's my favorite nurse. She brings me ice water when I get to the NICU and tells me to get more rest, which I appreciate. Just that little bit of empathy helps so much.

I don't know what I will do if Tenzin has a heart problem. I am trying not to blame myself, or to feel like I've failed somehow. Was it something I ate? Should I have gone to the "better" hospital? I never should have left Dr. Lowen. Glen tells me not to beat myself up, but when I see Tenzin lying there alone, or when I walk into the NICU and hear him screaming his heart out as doctors and nurses walk right by, it's almost impossible. Even if no one is to blame, still, someone has to show up and take responsibility. Someone has to apologize over and over, and hold him until he knows that, at the very least, it's not *his* fault.

December 30

We've been struggling with the breastfeeding. Tenzin has a good latch, but it is clearly difficult for him to breathe and nurse at the same time.

Now when he cries and wants to be fed, the nurses call me on the phone at two a.m., five a.m., eight a.m., eleven. Mommy Walker! Your baby is crying. Will you please come to feed him? I hear Tenzin screaming at the top of his lungs in the background and I leap out of bed, throw on my robe, and run over to give him some milk.

He drinks a little and then chokes, coughs, turns his head away. Between his breathing difficulty and the incredible amount of milk streaming out of my breasts, it might be too much. My breastfeeding book says that too much milk can overwhelm the baby and turn him off the breast completely. I spoke to Janet and she thinks I should stop pumping so often, to slow down the flow.

Now I'm anxious about traumatizing my baby with my breast milk! Glen thinks the bottle is the most manageable solution, but every time he suggests it I feel irrationally defensive. Last night I got really upset. I've already lost my postpartum bliss moment, I cried, now you want me to give up nursing, too? I am just so afraid we won't bond, or that he won't get what he needs, which is closeness with his mommy.

This afternoon a social worker came in to talk to us. I think she was trying to find out if there were any problems in our family like domestic abuse or drug addiction. She asked some very personal questions about our home life and told us about government programs we could apply for. Glen told me it was normal for the social worker to be available because the hospital is public and serves people who need help. She becomes their liaison.

I am glad of that, but she gave me the creeps. She started to give us a lecture on how different things were going to be with the baby and how we needed to prepare ourselves emotionally. I was like, Are you kidding?

I understand that people need services, but there was something not right about the approach, the assumptions made. Or maybe I just really want to go home with my baby and I am projecting my dissatisfaction onto the social worker.

The truth is, I am obscenely jealous of the mothers who have problem-free births. Their babies just hit the NICU to be cleaned off, weighed, and measured, and then it's right back up to mom. I caught myself today looking enviously at those babies and feeling sorry for myself and Tenzin.

December 31

The cardiac echo came back normal today. Whoopeee! He has been taken off fluids and is now just getting breast milk. He's finally gaining weight and Dr. Morales says he's looking good. Still not healing as fast as he should, but the fact that he's gained a few ounces is encouraging.

I needed the good news. Last night I beat myself up for hours for staying on the antidepressant; for being half in the medical model and half in the midwifery model; for being so consumed with my big ideas that something bad happened to my pure, innocent, faultless baby.

After Dr. Morales told me the good news, I walked the hospital halls drenched in relief. Where else could I go? Last night as I was agonizing over the barely detectable traces of antidepressant found in breast milk, Glen told me that I am too hard on myself. He's right. Cruising through the different wards, I decided that I'm just like every other mother. I want to do the right thing, but sometimes life doesn't work out the way I've planned.

January 1

Passed a quiet New Year's Eve in the NICU, holding Tenzin and looking into his inquisitive brown eyes. Already, in the brief moments he is actually awake, he studies everything about me. He is getting to know my outer terrain like he knew the inner one. When I walk through the glass door of the NICU, all I have to do is say loudly in his direction that I have arrived. He stops crying immediately and waits patiently for me to wash my hands. Then we do our ritual of getting the pillow right, and my glass of water within reach, and the little stool under my feet. I lift him without pulling his monitor leads off and pop my bra open at the same time, sidle him up to my breast, and then we are off on the magic carpet ride.

Happy New Year, sweet and precious boy. I am so glad you made it.

January 2

Does being a mother mean that your heart is cracked open forever?

This morning as I was feeding Tenzin, I noticed the nurses packing baby Christopher up to leave. I was interested because while I have been keeping my eye on Christopher, a delicate, quiet baby with seemingly no complications, I had never seen his mom. I figured that our schedules were just off, but this morning I realized it wasn't that at all. His mom left him here the day he was born.

The nurses packed all he had—a few diapers, a box of wipes, some bottles, and his little name card—while a foster mother waited in the hallway. I had seen her, the woman who was going to be Christopher's first love, on my way to the NICU. She was older, and looked tired and overwhelmed. She had a teenager with her, a boy, probably another foster child.

I could hardly stand it. Here I've been so worried about Tenzin and all he doesn't have. When I asked, Rose told me that

Christopher's mother was a drug addict who had given birth
here before. A discussion about birth control for drug-addicted
women ensued, but I couldn't join in. I had to will myself to stay
in my chair holding my baby, instead of getting on the phone to
marshal resources for Christopher. Could we bring him home?
Who did I know who wanted a baby? I was sure I could find a
nice gay couple that would shower him with love.

But of course, I did nothing. There was nothing for me to do.
Baby Christopher was bundled and handed to a complete
stranger. I will never know if he ever laid eyes on the woman
who made him, but I will always wonder.

RAINY DAY. I spent it cleaning my new room here at the hospital, finishing shower thank-you notes, and nursing Tenzin. Felt a
bit melancholy. Something about the light, and being here in the
city. Glen came with bags and bags of food to restock the cooler
he set up for me. We sat on the little green sofa, looking out at the
rain and eating tangerines.

January 5

I took a taxi from the hospital to get my toes painted, because I
needed to get out of the hospital and return, just for a moment, to
life as I once knew it. I put on my black pregnancy pants, battered
denim shirt, and a little lip gloss, and left Glen sound asleep in the
hospital bed with his head and feet up. The moment I stepped off
the elevator and saw people in their everyday clothes, going about
their lives, I started to feel out of sync. The world looked exactly

as it did before, but I felt completely different. The dissonance made everything seem surreal. I kept telling myself that I have survived the act of bringing a child into the world and am in the process of surviving the fight to keep him alive. But there weren't any billboards up for that.

I showed up at the salon with my hospital bracelets, the plastic strips that verify that I actually do have a child in the NICU, around my wrist. Because babies are often abducted from hospitals, nurses in the NICU must match the numbers on my band to the ones on Tenzin's. If the numbers are not the same, or if I don't have a band at all, the nurses are required, no matter what I say or how loudly my baby is crying, to restrict my access. I hadn't paid much attention to them, but outside of the hospital they're pretty noticeable. Yelena spotted them right away and raised her eyebrows when I walked into the salon. I told her the baby's fine, just having a bit of trouble breathing.

When I finally got my feet into the hot water, I asked Raya why she didn't warn me. I had a smile on my face, but I was serious, too. Why didn't anybody tell me how much it was going to hurt? There were a few nodding heads, and then Raya said, I know, I know. It's awful. And I said, You know? Where were you, where was everybody, when I was talking all that natural-childbirth shit? Someone should have told me that I was out of my mind and that it was like getting a root canal without anesthetic.

After an hour and a half of being out, I started to miss the baby like crazy. My breasts were leaking through the pads in my bra, and I felt an overwhelming need to get back to the hospital.

It lifted me out of the chair and out of the salon and into a taxi and back to the hospital. It didn't stop until I flashed my wristband at the nurse, walked through the door of the NICU, and saw with my own eyes that my baby was alive. Still breathing through a tube strapped to his face, but alive.

January 9

Went out for a walk today with Glen. When we got back to the hospital, the security guards had Tenzin's name but not mine on their chart. I flashed my hospital I.D. bracelets a few times, and tried to calmly explain the situation, you know, that the baby is sick and I am rooming in, but they refused to let me up.

I don't know exactly what happened, but Glen says I turned into some kind of Warrior Woman. I remember that when I realized they were serious and not planning to let me up, I felt a sharp surge of energy and also a preternatural calm. Everything got quiet and still. I wasn't sure how it would go down, but it occurred to me that if these guys didn't change their minds about letting me upstairs to see my baby, I couldn't guarantee their safety.

I think I told them that I didn't care what their chart said, my baby was upstairs and I was going to see him, but I remember that I made a sharp gesture with my hands. I remember that afterward they both stepped back and let us pass. I remember everything being quiet until the elevator door closed in front of us. Then Glen made a joke about me being a superhero. He said as we were walking toward the elevator all he could think was, *I'm with her.*

We were still laughing about it hours later, likening it to the Star Wars moment when the Storm Troopers stop Obi-Wan and demand his identification. Obi-Wan waves his hand over their faces and says, "You don't need to see my identification," and they magically parrot back to him, "We don't need your identification," and let him and Luke pass unmolested.

It's now official. The Force they're talking about? It's the cosmic version of motherhood.

January 13

He's been off oxygen for six hours, with the cannula still in place. Everyone keeps checking on him to see how he's doing and telling me we'll be going home soon. Rose told me today that they've done all they can do for him here. It's time for him to go home and live. She keeps saying in that singsongy voice, Mr. Tenzeen, you are going home, Mr. Tenzeen. And then she pinches his cheeks and smiles.

Glen and I spoke to Dr. Thompson, who is authorizing his release tomorrow barring any major sat dips. He stressed that Tenzin was probably going to be one-hundred-percent fine, able to do everything a kid who hadn't had MAS could do. The difficulty, he said, would be his parents treating him like a sick kid all his life. That's the tendency, he said. Mothers and fathers, but mostly mothers, fretting over kids who have been sick, telling them they shouldn't do this and shouldn't do that, and projecting weak, sick child ideas all over them.

They were speaking in guyese about overprotective mothers,

smothers. I was about to get pissed and vehemently deny that I would ever be that way, but then I thought I heard Tenzin's monitor beeping and ran over to make sure he was okay. Clearly, I've got to take baby steps.

The biggest news is that the baby is going to sleep with me tonight! I can't believe it. The experience we've all been waiting for. After dinner, if he makes it without the cannula for three hours, one of the nurses is going to wheel him into my room and we get to be there together for the entire night. No tubes, no machines, no constant in-and-out of doctors and other parents. Just us: my boy and me, in the quiet dark.

January 14

It was hard to say goodbye to everybody, but easy to leave the hospital. I hugged and thanked all the nurses I could find. I accepted and read the card wishing Tenzin a happy and success-ful life, signed by all of the doctors. I collected all fourteen bottles of my breast milk from the refrigerator and put them in a cooler bought expressly, no pun intended, for this purpose.

Angie wheeled us downstairs as Glen pulled up in the big car we bought for just this moment. After much wrestling with straps, I settled Tenzin in his new seat.

Within seconds we were on the freeway and the hospital was far behind us. Glen put his hand over mine and I felt the warmth of it, of him, radiate through my whole body. I thought about how Glen had showed up for me and we had showed up for Ten-zin. And I thought that really, when it comes down to it, that's what life is all about: showing up for the people you love, again and again, until you can't show up anymore.

I put my hand over his and said, We did it. We made a baby and now we are taking him home.

Glen looked at me and said, Yep. I think that about covers it.

And then we laughed.

Nine

LIKE EVERY OTHER warm-blooded woman of childbearing age, I worried a great deal about the many wonderful experiences I would have to forgo once I had a baby. Along with sleep, travel, and ready-to-wear, movies were at the top of my list of things I simply could not imagine life without. New and old, foreign and domestic, comedies, dramas, and documentaries: I watched them tucked cozily into bed at night, or lounging on the sofa in the early morning. They were like chocolate to me: delicious, transporting, and essential.

Now I can't believe I watched so many movies. When I go down the list of films on Netflix, I am appalled by how hard it is to find one I haven't seen. How many hours of my life have I spent on long, artfully drawn journeys into other people's lives? Human beings crave narrative because we glimpse the universal through the specific and feel less alone. But I feel nothing but relief to be so fully occupied living my own life that I am no longer compelled to watch other people living theirs.

Call me a snob, but where I used to find the infinite ways people resolve their endlessly complicated lives fascinating, I now see a bunch of stylized variations on a theme. It's not that storytelling or art itself isn't valuable, because it irrefutably is. I couldn't bring myself to write this book if it wasn't. I am just newly aware that it may not be *absolutely necessary*. I can have a perfectly fulfilling life, without entering the mind-streams of dozens of artists trying to make sense of their temporal existence. This feels blasphemous to think, let alone write, but I have to be brutally honest here, because that's my job.

I had a baby and yes, I am like every new mother in that all I want to do is stare at him all day. But beneath that desire is a more profound truth: *He* is the story! The fact that he's here, that he's mine, and that anything could happen to either of us. The incontrovertible truth that he materialized miraculously: a flesh-and-blood manifestation of a figment of my imagination, and that I have to work like hell to subject him to all of the yummy and none of the yucky stuff of my own childhood.

In this new live-it-or-leave-it modality, I realize I may be flirting dangerously with myopia, and that it could be a stage, like teething, that will pass. I may wake up one morning rabid for a trip to the multiplex, but I don't think so. The transition from observer to participant has been inexplicably liberating. It's the how-to-live-your-own-life version of learning to swim: Once you know how, you no longer need lessons. You just get in the ocean and go.

This, I'll call it "life competence" for lack of a better term, is permeating my life. Now when I am lusting after a pair of boots, I have to ask myself if I'll be wearing those to the decidedly unglamorous supermarket down the street to pick up diapers and sliced turkey, and whether or not the toe will be a help or a hindrance when it's time to unfold the stroller. When I consider yet another price tag, for anything, I am forced to consider how much interest the same amount of money would earn in a 529 college savings plan.

I can't say that I am completely sober, but the whole process, that holy trinity of hunt, acquisition, and display, is breaking down as my concern shifts from looking great and feeling slightly alienated to feeling incredible and looking relatively well-put-together. Instead of talking through "stuff," I am talking to my son. I am not saying a girl can't have it all, because I am all for making life expand to meet your limitless vision, but I am saying that, first, said girl has to know what "all" really is.

My work habits have also taken a turn. A few days ago, a friend with writer's block asked about my favorite places to write. Was it the desert or the forest, a spa or hotel, a lonely retreat cabin or a convivial writers' colony? Struck by the question, I flashed on all the climates and landscapes I have pursued in the name of writing, all the rooms and houses, offices and shacks I've spent months and years trying to transform into the perfect writing space. Where did it get me? Where is my bookshelf filled with titles?

I didn't want to shatter the hopeful promise of the room of one's own, that mystical and magical place the muse will be unable to resist, but again, I had to tell the truth.

My bed, I said. My dining-room table, the tiny thirty-dollar

desk on casters I bought at IKEA, the sofa. At the moment, I am
writing at the kitchen table. Tenzin is strapped into his carrot-
encrusted high chair on my right, engrossed in picking up star-
shaped banana puffs. Every five minutes, he makes a high-pitched
yelp to get my attention, and I reach for a new thrill to keep
him occupied, but by the end of the day I will have written five
hundred words over my thousand-word allotment. As an extra
bonus, I get to sneak a quick kiss or neck nuzzle in between
graphs.

My friend was taken aback, but not after I explained that
writing-room obsession had claimed many years of actual writing time; that the cultivation of the perfect space was my procras-
tination activity of choice. I told her that back when I was
searching for the ideal space, I'd be lucky if I even turned on my
computer, let alone banged out a few lines. I probably will never
catch up to Stephen King, who at a professed eighty to eighty-five
pages a day makes me sick with envy, but now I am closer than
ever to writing a book a year, and I owe it all to Tenzin.

Of course, it's not all chocolate and roses over here. Yesterday
I heard from one of my cousins that he has replaced me in my
mother's will. I can only assume that her response to my request
for an apology is to disinherit me. It hurts, but she's been talking
for so many years about how she doesn't believe in leaving anything to one's children, I am numb to it. Of course, now that I have
a child and can't watch the evening news without wondering how
on earth any of us are going to survive, I can't imagine not wanting
to take care of my children and my children's children.

I also got a call from the caretaker of the little house in Mendocino I spent so much time transforming. He told me that my

mother told him to throw all of my clothes and belongings away. *Todo,* he said. *¡En la basura!* The truth is that what my mother is doing hurts so much I can no longer feel it, but I am more confident than ever about my decision to keep my distance. It's not just me now getting yanked about by her anger and ambivalence, her refusal to acknowledge my right to my own story, it's Tenzin, too. All these years I haven't been able to stand up for myself, but now, for him, I'm willing to walk through fire. Which is about what becoming a mother without a mother feels like.

There are other complications, too. Like all the things I miss—sleep, for example. When people told me to rest while I was pregnant, I didn't know what to think. I'm an eight-hour-a-night person, and I figured I might have to settle for six. Not two to four, interrupted every forty-five minutes by piercing screams, hurried bottle preparation, and hushed whispers to a disoriented creature in a padded box. Not so little sleep that I would be rendered virtually incompetent physically, emotionally, and in tens of other ways I am too tired to remember.

I miss being able to wander aimlessly, not knowing the time, not caring, not having to phone home to make sure baby boy isn't having a ballistic fit. Being "responsible" for my time is undeniably a mark of my growing appreciation for its value, but God damn, it's hell. These days, if I am on my own I am either on the clock paying by the hour, or feeling guiltily beholden to my wonderful but sometimes overwhelmed partner who has his own work to do. Naptime, no matter how much I want to believe is free time, is not. I can't go out of earshot, and must be ready to stop whatever I am doing to attend to the babe. Gone are my two-hour mini-vacations in the bathtub.

I miss my breasts, which, while still perfectly lovely and functional, have definitely gone through some changes since per-
forming their duties as organic milk dispensers. I miss my flat
stomach. It's coming back slowly, but I have the sinking suspicion
it will never be the same. I miss having what felt like an endless
supply of mental and emotional stamina. Where I used to seek out
conversation, licking my lips at the possibility of a "meaningful
exchange," I am increasingly more selective about how I expend
my precious energy.

And even though loving another human being a thousand
times more than you love yourself is arguably the most subver-
sive thrill left in this object-obsessed, hypercapitalist world, I
miss having only myself to worry about. The constant fear for
my baby's psychological and physical well-being is noble, but
enervating in every way.

Even so, as I consider the fact that I, once terrified of spiders,
will now reach into my son's crib to kill one with my bare hands,
I am struck by the human ability—propensity, even—for regen-
eration and change. It's true that we are what we think, but the
caveat is that what we think changes, and thank goodness. If we
weren't gradually disabused of limited ideas about the world and
ourselves, who would we be? Five years ago I thought I could
find marital bliss with an unfaithful musician, and happiness in a
house renovation. Ten years ago, I thought meat was murder and
meat eaters should be forced to raise and slaughter their own
suppers. Thirteen years ago, I thought I was going to marry a
devout Muslim and raise ten kids on a tiny island with no running water or electricity.

That we can change our minds is the easy part, it's figuring

out what to change them to that is nearly impossible. I suggest an identity, or should I say a series of decisions, that make one happy and ensure the psychological well-being of the next generation. Isn't that the ultimate freedom? To know you're serving yourself and the present while at the same time taking care of the future?

I am a mother and a partner now. After all those years of wanting, denying, and being afraid, I stopped searching and embraced what was right in front of me. It's hard, this making a healthy family, probably the hardest work I've ever done. But every day, when I look at this little being I have the extreme good fortune to call my son, I thank the part of me that had the where-withal, despite all the doubt and fear, to go ahead and embrace motherhood, to get on the ride and let it take me away.

I have no regrets.

ACKNOWLEDGMENTS

Everyone needs a team, and I feel blessed to have one so loyal and devoted.

Thanks to my literary agent, Jennifer Rudolph Walsh, for being one of the toughest, smartest women I've ever known and for having my back. Thanks to Geoff Kloske and Sarah McGrath for leading the Riverhead charge with insight and grace, and for making this a better book. Thanks to Amy Hertz and Cindy Spiegel, who have moved on but are not forgotten. Thanks, again, to Susan Petersen Kennedy.

Thanks to Barbara Wilson and Alba Camarena for funding my SEP IRA. Thanks to Aurélie Moulin for keeping my virtual world beautiful and up-to-date. Thanks to Ekajati Moore for orchestrating my day-to-day with élan. Thanks to all of the lecture agents that keep me comfortable on the road.

Thanks to my father, for always trying to find integrity no

matter how difficult the circumstances. Thanks to my mother for having the courage to live her truth and, by example, teaching me to live mine. Thanks to Randall and Nicole for being there through it all.

Finally, thanks to all the readers who find meaning in my work.

You make it all worthwhile.

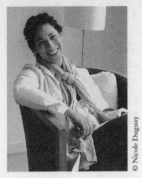

© Nicole Duguay

ABOUT THE AUTHOR

Named by *Time* magazine as one of the most influential leaders of her generation, Rebecca Walker has received numerous awards and accolades for her writing and activism, including the Alex Award from the American Library Association and an honorary doctorate from the North Carolina School of the Arts. In addition to the bestselling memoir *Black, White, and Jewish,* she is the editor of the anthologies *To Be Real: Telling the Truth and Changing the Face of Feminism,* a standard text in gender studies courses around the world, and *What Makes a Man: 22 Writers Imagine the Future.* Please visit her at www.rebeccawalker.com.

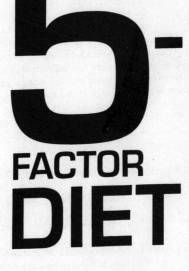

THE
5-
FACTOR
DIET

Harley Pasternak, M. Sc.,

with Myatt Murphy

Ballantine Books ╟╫╫╢ New York

Author's Note: This book is intended to provide helpful guidance and information on the subject of diet and exercise; it is not meant to be taken as medical advice or to replace the diagnostic expertise of a physician. You should aways refer any questions or concerns about your health to a trusted medical professional, particularly if you are pregnant, nursing an infant, or suffering from any medical condition or symptom. As with any diet or exercise program, stop immediately and consult a doctor if you experience pain or discomfort at any time.

2009 Ballantine Books Trade Paperback Edition

Copyright © 2006 by Harley Pasternak

All rights reserved.

Published in the United States by Ballantine Books, an imprint of The Random House Publishing Group, a division of Random House, Inc., New York.

BALLANTINE and colophon are registered trademarks of Random House, Inc.

Originally published in hardcover in the United States by Meredith Books in 2006.

ISBN 978-0-345-51349-6

Library of Congress Control Number: 2006930029

Printed in the United States of America

www.ballantinebooks.com

2 4 6 8 9 7 5 3 1

This book is dedicated to all my clients.
You have been, and continue to be, my
guinea pigs, my inspiration, and my friends.

ACKNOWLEDGMENTS

My parents. To whom I owe all my success.

My brothers, Jesse and Bobby. My best friends and my fountain of youth.

My manager, Kristin Giese. I treasure your leadership and strength.

My literary agent, Andrea Barzvi. The only agent I will ever have.

My cowriter, Myatt Murphy. For sharing my vision and being so professional.

My editor, Stephanie Karpinske. For polishing the words.

Paola Patrella. For your delicious recipes.

Logan Alexander. For your photography and humor.

Carmen Bonicci. My Canadian strategist.

My commercial agent, Brittany Balbo, for your support.

My closest friends, Dave, Anne, Behzad, Sam, Rachel, Wendy, Michael, David, Jamie, Ricky, Jeff, Josh, David, Rick, John, Brian, Jen, Jodi, Vera, and Wil. For reminding me where I'm from and who I am.

Lucy and Viv. You are always in my heart.

Contents

This book took me 15 years to write.

Not really 15 years of writing ... more like a decade and a half of evolution.

The 5-Factor evolution started when I was a "husky" teenager ("husky" is simply a kinder way of saying overweight). I bought every diet book, fitness magazine, and exotic weight loss pill, powder, and bar! I tried weight training, step aerobics classes, Pilates, and yoga. I experimented with diets such as Pritikin, Body For Life, and the Zone. I became interested in exercise and nutrition as a way to make me look and feel better. However, it wasn't until both of my younger brothers were diagnosed with type 1 diabetes that I became interested in the science of food and how it affects our bodies. I spent eight years in university studying metabolism, biochemistry, nutrition, and physiology. I call this period my "nerd years."

While I was in graduate school, the 5-Factor evolution continued as I began to work as a nutrition scientist for the Canadian Department of National Defense. I learned a great deal about research. Not only did I perform my own nutrition studies (breaking many test tubes in the process), but I also learned how to assess existing nutrition research. Equipped with studies that could definitively support or refute popular diet info, I began to question many dietary practices. I thought more critically about claims I heard about popular diet programs and weight loss supplements.

I reread all the diet books I had previously treated as gospel and underlined all of the "facts" the books used to support their claims. I then set out to find the research these claims were based on. To my chagrin, I realized most diets and weight loss strategies are quick-fix programs based on half-truths and flat-out fabrications.

I knew there had to be a way of eating healthy that would also be realistic. I wanted a program based on real truth, real science, and real people's lifestyles, a sensible system that would promote fat loss *and* enjoyment.

My 5-Factor evolution continued as my nutrition and fitness practice grew. I developed and refined my nutrition plan and applied it to clients with amazing results. My program garnered the attention of actors who wanted to tone up for upcoming roles. Nineteen films, nine television shows, and more than 50 actor and musician clients later, my 5-Factor Diet has helped the likes of Halle Berry, Alicia Keys, Kanye West, Mandy Moore, Eva Mendes, Rachel Weisz, Rick Fox, John Mayer, Brendan Fraser, Stephen Dorff, Robert Downey Jr., and Benjamin Bratt.

In 2005 my first book, *5-Factor Fitness*, hit the top of two bestseller lists. Though *5-Factor Fitness* was primarily an exercise plan, it contained a brief introduction to the 5-Factor Diet and offered a number of quick 5-Factor recipes. I received more than 5,000 emails from people who had purchased *5-Factor Fitness* and had shed anywhere from 5 to 87 pounds! Nearly all of them requested more 5-Factor recipes and wanted to know more about the 5-Factor Diet.

So, with great pride, I present you with the last diet book you will ever purchase. Welcome to *The 5-Factor Diet*.

Harley Pasternak, M.Sc.

CHAPTER 1

A Fresh Start

We've met before.

I don't know your name or where you live, but it's safe to say that I do know you—and I know why you're reading this book.

You're not happy with your body.

It doesn't matter whether you're looking to drop a few pounds, firm up, or improve your health so you can live a longer life; all of these goals start with eating right.

Most likely you've already tried some—it probably seems like *all*—of the different diets that are popular today. It's likely that you even lost some weight. But if you're like most people, you gained some or all of it back. Or worse, you regained it all plus a few extra pounds. You're sick and tired of fighting the "fat war," running caloric calculations in your head and denying yourself entire food groups. You're fed up with weighing your food at every meal, scrimping on portions, and eating tasteless diet foods while salivating over the cooking shows on TV—all in an effort to look as lean, fit, and glamorous as the movie stars you admire on the big screen.

Well, I have some news for you. Television actors and movie stars don't make the same mistakes that you have. And with the 5-Factor Diet, you won't make those mistakes ever again. Absolutely anyone can get into better shape quickly—the harder part, of course, is staying that way. 5-Factor can help.

MY HOLLYWOOD SECRETS ARE NOW YOURS

When my first book, 5-Factor Fitness, became an overnight success in 2005, I was proud that the system I've been using for years with my Hollywood clients was finally available to everyone. In the book I outlined a 5-week program to jump-start readers to a better body and healthier lifestyle, focusing primarily on fitness and exercise.

Since the book was published, I've been overwhelmed with requests from readers like you asking for more information on diet and nutrition. The sheer volume of letters I've received has made it clear to me that people want to know more about the nutritional plan I use with my clients—particularly the 5-minute meals that are part of my program—and how to incorporate it into their day-to-day lives.

The 5-Factor Diet book you're holding is my new nutritional bible, a complete guide to the simple yet extraordinarily effective diet program I've used for years with my celebrity clients to get them—and keep them—in great shape.

My 5-Factor Diet stands alone as a nutritional program that is simple yet comprehensive. More important, it actually works. Having this book on your shelf will be like having your very own round-the-clock personal nutritionist and chef on hand. It's the result of my many years of education and experience in the weight loss industry, with proven results you can see anytime one of my celebrity clients makes a movie, strolls down the red carpet, or poses for a magazine. The 5-Factor Diet is not just another diet book. I promise, this will be the last diet book you'll ever need.

THE 5-FACTOR DIET

So why do I call my program the 5-Factor Diet? That's easy! Or, I should say, it's to make things easier for you. Every nutritional and

"I suffered from extremely poor health and almost died twice within the same year, a situation that left me too sick and unable to exercise for over three years. I had no energy and I gave up exercise altogether until I tried 5-Factor. The simplicity of the plan and, more important, seeing amazingly quick results made it easy for me to stay dedicated to the program. It's magic!"

Louise Meinardus AGE: **40s** WEIGHT LOST SO FAR: **5 lbs.**

exercise principle I'm about to teach you breaks down into five easy-to-remember points:

+ The 5-Factor Diet is a 5-week diet plan.
+ There are 5 types of food you should eat in every meal.
+ The Diet incorporates a 5-phase 5-Factor Hollywood Workout.
+ My exercise routine, like my diet, is simple: 5 workouts a week, each consisting of five 5-minute phases.
+ To follow my diet, you'll want to try some of my 100-plus 5-Factor recipes, which require only 5 (or fewer) main ingredients. Each delicious recipe can be prepared in 5 minutes or less. (That doesn't count cooking time, of course; I said delicious, not miraculous!)

I promise: If you can count to 5, the 5-Factor Diet will be the easiest diet you'll ever use to lose.

YOU'RE READY TO START!
Before I get into detail about the simplicity and effectiveness of the 5-Factor Diet—and teach you the scientific basis for it—I want to talk to you about all the fad diets you may have tried in the past. Because you can't move forward without figuring out why you've been falling

backward, it's important to understand why every other diet has ultimately failed you. Turn the page to finally break yourself of the yo-yo
diet cycle forever.

Sophia Bush ACTRESS, STAR OF THE TV HIT *ONE TREE HILL*

*"To me, Harley's plan is an eating and fitness
plan that makes sense, allows me to eat
real food, and gives me compact, effective
workouts. I actually crave a healthy lifestyle.
It feels incredible!"*

CHAPTER 2

Fad Diets Don't Work

A client came to me about 40 pounds overweight and frustrated. Over the three preceding years, he had lost 200 pounds, desperately trying a variety of fad diets. Sounds impressive, right?

It wasn't.

When I say he lost 200 pounds, that's counting the weight he had lost and gained back. He would drop 40 pounds, then gain 50 back. He would lose 50 pounds, then gain 60 back! It's called yo-yo dieting or weight cycling. It's not just a waste of your time; it could do your body harm.

Today's fad diets are merely the latest in a long line of ineffective and often dangerous diet crazes. Over the past 20 years, Americans have been bombarded with one diet after another. Though the diets appear to be as different from each other as night and day, they all have something in common: They only work *up to a certain point*, if they work at all.

I believe that once you understand why these diets fall short, you can choose a more sensible plan and achieve the body and healthy lifestyle you've always hoped for. I don't want you to waste any more time or effort on diets that won't work. Failure is something your body simply can't afford.

In doing research for the 5-Factor Diet, I read dozens of diet books. As someone who makes a living educating people about health and fitness, I was shocked at how ridiculous many of these diets were.

You see, whenever you begin a low-calorie diet, your body notices that it's being fed fewer calories and immediately lowers your basal metabolic rate (BMR)—the rate at which your body burns calories. That means the result of eating fewer calories is burning fewer calories all day long. Once you quit the diet—and you will—it takes a while for your body to bring your BMR back to normal.

That's why yo-yo dieters end up gaining more and more weight with each diet failure. If you go back to your old eating habits while your BMR is still low, you won't just regain the pounds you lost, you'll pack a few extra on top. Repeat this cycle a few times and you end up gaining more weight the more often you try to lose it. It's physically exhausting and emotionally frustrating.

I want you to ask yourself what I consider the single most important health and fitness question: Do you want to look good tomorrow or do you want to look good for the rest of your life?

You need to think of your health and fitness goals as a marathon instead of a sprint. Most fad diets claim they can help you drop pounds fast, and I know that promise can be incredibly alluring. But that weight loss is usually the result of nutritional tactics that are not only unhealthy but also impossible to maintain.

To take pounds off for good, it's all about finishing the race. You need an effective and efficient plan of attack that lets you lose weight consistently, not just immediately. What differentiates the 5-Factor Diet from all the fad diets that I'm about to discuss is this: While all of these fad diets work for a short time, only the 5-Factor Diet will keep you lean and healthy for a lifetime.

BLOOD TYPE DIET

This diet claims it's your blood type, not just the calories you consume, that causes weight gain. According to the program, the secret to losing fat is to eat only specific foods that are compatible with your blood type. Eating the wrong foods is supposedly like receiving a transfusion of the wrong type of blood, causing substances from your food, called lectins, to enter your bloodstream. It's this flow of lectins that supposedly causes blood cells to clot, leading to a variety of health issues.

The diet's claims about blood type and weight loss are not backed up by relevant scientific research. Your blood type has nothing to do with your body's ability to burn excess fat. The plan restricts not only calories but food types as well. You're told not to eat certain healthy foods that are rich in antioxidants, vitamins, and minerals. And the diet recommends some unusual foods and supplements that are only available online.

CABBAGE SOUP DIET

It's easy to see why so many people have tried this strict, low-calorie program that has been around for decades. Its proponents claim you can drop up to 20 pounds in seven days by eating little more than cabbage-based soup several times a day. Cycling on and off the diet (7 days on, 14 days off) is said to promote rapid weight loss.

This diet can be harmful to your body because it restricts your caloric intake to less than 1,000 calories a day. It leaves you feeling perpetually hungry because you're basically forcing your body to live off nothing but fiber and water. There's no protein or fats and few vitamins or minerals. The weight loss most people see is almost always water and lean muscle mass because the lack of protein causes your body to cannibalize its own muscle tissue. You will also likely have uncomfortable side effects such as diarrhea, abdominal pain, light-headedness, and flatulence.

GRAPEFRUIT DIET

In this popular diet, you're required to eat a whole grapefruit with every meal. Why a grapefruit? According to the diet, grapefruits contain a special fat-burning enzyme.

The negatives of this diet are identical to those of the Cabbage Soup Diet, even though the plan does allow small amounts of protein. It's not the grapefruit that deserves the credit for whatever weight is lost; this restrictive, 800-calorie diet basically starves you. No matter how much you may wish otherwise, there is simply no such thing as a superfood with magical abilities to make you lose weight.

CAVEMAN DIET

The creators of this nutrition plan believe that cavemen and cavewomen were lean and healthy because of the all-natural foods they ate. According to this diet, processed and cultivated foods, including wheat and grains, are the true cause of all major disease and obesity. The diet requires you to return to your Neanderthal roots by eating only what your ancestors did. That means eliminating all processed foods in favor of natural foods such as fish, lean meats, berries, vegetables, fruits, nuts, and seeds.

I can't argue with the premise that the less processed a food is, the healthier it is for your body. However, it is a stretch to claim that the lack of processed foods was the main reason our ancestors were leaner than we are. But they also had to spend many physically demanding hours hunting down or picking their own food.

Cavemen were so lean in part because they were much more physically active than we are today. Yet that factor is never considered in the caveman equation. Nor does the diet discuss the fact that our ancestors lacked convenient access to food and thus ate significantly less than we do. And there is no scientific research to date that links wheat or grains to obesity and resulting diseases—yet this diet claims that corn is responsible for more cancer deaths than cigarettes. There is a more logical reason why our ancestors didn't suffer from cancer, heart disease, and other

"I tried practically every fad diet invented, but they never worked long term. The 5-Factor Diet opened my eyes to correct, healthy eating. By following Harley's plan, I was finally able to learn to change my eating habits. Diets come and go, but Harley's plan is for the rest of your life!"

Danielle Martin AGE: 37 WEIGHT LOST SO FAR: 77 lbs.

Sanaa Lathan ACTRESS AND STAR OF THE MOVIE *LOVE AND BASKETBALL*

"I was asked to lose some weight for my last film. Harley had me do his 5-Factor Diet and exercise program. Within weeks my body was transformed. Getting in shape was never this easy. And I just saw my movie. And if I may say so myself, my body looks better than it ever has on film. I'm a fan for life."

modern-day ailments: They never grew old because the average life span of a Neanderthal man was 20 years!

NO SUGAR DIET

This diet eliminates foods that are high in refined sugar and carbohydrates that rank high on the glycemic index.

Break out your calculator because you'll have to make sure every meal is divided into 30 percent carbohydrates, 30 percent protein, and 40 percent fat. Not only are these calculations time-consuming, but your daily caloric consumption is limited to an unhealthy 1,200 calories. You don't lose weight because you're eating less sugar; you lose it because you're eating too few calories. The diet restricts many healthy-for-you foods, such as carrots, that contain ample amounts of essential vitamins and minerals. Instead, it claims you can lose weight while eating high-fat, low-sugar foods such as hamburger, steak, and cheese.

LIQUID DIETS

These diets make you forgo food in favor of a liquid meal replacement drink typically made from sugar, fat-free milk powder, fiber, vitamins, and minerals. On some versions of the plan you eat only shakes; on others you also have small, low-calorie meals.

One of my clients was on a shake diet for a while. Every day she drank five shakes instead of eating real food. She was miserable and depressed, especially when she went out to dinner at a five-star restaurant and had to bring a shake with her instead of eating the delicious meals.

Liquid diets are antisocial, and they're not sustainable because they're not satisfying. Research has shown that liquids don't fill your stomach as effectively as solid foods. And most of these shakes are deficient in dietary fiber, so you never feel quite as full. These low-calorie diets—as low as 700 calories—can stress your kidneys because many liquid dieters end up dehydrated.

NEW BEVERLY HILLS DIET

This diet has you combine foods in particular ways in order to create a certain mix of enzymes that supposedly helps your body properly digest your food.

Although combining certain types of foods can be beneficial for losing weight—something I'll explain later as part of the 5-Factor Diet—but it's not because of the enyme mix in food, as this diet claims. The truth is, the enzymes used to digest food are created by your body.

The theory that any food that can't be digested properly "adds" weight doesn't make sense either. If your body can't break down food, that means it has less chance to grab the calories and store them as body fat. Regardless of theories, this diet is also too low in protein, vitamins, and minerals to be considered healthy.

BODY FOR LIFE

This is a six-day-a-week diet and exercise plan whose creator promises that you'll be in the best shape of your life after 12 weeks.

You'll notice that Body For Life encourages you to use a lot of nutritional supplements. In fact, the program seems to be designed mainly to sell these supplements. One thing I do approve of about the Body For Life plan is that it encourages regular exercise.

HIGH-FIBER DIETS

The theory behind super-high-fiber diets is that if you overeat fibrous foods, your meals travel through your digestive system at an accelerated

> "Your book turned my life around after 15 years away from the gym had taken its toll. It was exactly what I needed to get back on track! I started using 5-Factor when I weighed 250 pounds and had a 42-inch waist. I am currently 185 pounds with a 32-inch waist. I feel amazing! Your book has given me the desire and discipline to attain a physical goal I thought was part of my past and never to be seen again!"
>
> **Andrew White** AGE: **39** WEIGHT LOST SO FAR: **65 lbs.**

pace, preventing your body from absorbing all the calories.

Eating fiber daily offers many health benefits. But eating excessive amounts of fiber doesn't guarantee weight loss. Fiber has no absorbable calories, which simply means that high-fiber diets are lower in calories. That's the real reason you lose weight initially on these diets.

However, eating excessive amounts of fiber can be rough on the digestive system. And it may push healthy, nutrient-rich foods out of your system with the fiber, preventing nutrients from being absorbed.

ORNISH PLAN AND PRITIKIN DIET

The Ornish plan limits your protein intake to a mere 15 percent of your total daily calories. It also claims that any calories from fat cause you to get fat. The Pritikin diet forces you to limit fat consumption to less than 10 percent of your total daily calories.

With such low amounts of protein (Ornish plan) or fat (Pritikin diet), it's not likely that you'll feel full on either diet. That's why some people overeat on these plans or can't stick to the program for any great length of time.

POINT PLANS AND PREPARED MEALS

Some weight loss plans limit the amount you eat by assigning you points based on your body weight and weight loss goals. The challenge with that is if you're not careful, you can gobble up all your points in one or two meals. That may leave you starving later in the day.

There are also diet plans that require you to buy packaged meals. On these plan, dieters often find themselves at a loss for what to eat when they aren't at home because they're not taught how to create their own healthy meals. Plus these plans can be pricey. Chances are, it's your bank account that will decide when you quit.

CHAPTER 3

Low-Carb Diets Don't Work

I believe that low-carbohydrate, high-protein diets, such as the Atkins diet, the South Beach Diet, and the Zone Diet, are as unhealthy and dangerous as any fad diet. But because they have been immensely popular for the past decade, I feel they deserve a chapter of their own.

So what is a high-protein, low-carb diet? It's any diet that stresses eating lots of protein (such as meat and eggs) while severely limiting carbohydrates (such as bread, potatoes, pasta, and rice). Most low-carb diets also make you avoid fruits, vegetables, and other good-for-you foods.

WHAT YOU LOSE—BESIDES WEIGHT—ON THESE DIETS

What's made low-carb diets so popular is that you do drop off pounds—at least in the short term. But instead of losing fat, these are the five things you're losing on a low-carb diet.

1. WATER

Although low-carb, high-protein diets cause a sudden weight loss initially, much of what you're losing is water. When you starve yourself of carbs, your body is left with no choice but to use up its glycogen, which is the stored carbohydrates it keeps on reserve to fuel activity. Each gram of glycogen has 3 to 4 grams of water attached to it, so as your body uses it up, excess water is shed, and the needle on the scale starts to move downward. The problem is, as soon as you go back to eating normally, your body restocks glycogen—and the excess water—so the weight comes right back.

2. MUSCLE

After its initial water-weight loss, your body has to turn elsewhere to find calories to fuel activity. That's when it starts gobbling up any lean muscle and organ tissue it can find as a source of energy.

3. NUTRIENTS AND FIBER

Most low-carb diets limit the amount of fresh fruits and vegetables you can eat. This leaves your body severely deficient in vitamins and minerals, not to mention dietary fiber.

4. INTEREST

Because so many foods (fruits, cereals, breads, grains, starches, baked goods, dairy products, starchy vegetables, and sweets) are eliminated or severely limited, this kind of diet is very hard to incorporate into life on a long-term basis. After a few weeks of following any low-carb regime, you'll lose interest in the diet because you're constantly feeling hungry and unsatisfied with the food you're allowed to eat.

5. YOUR HEALTH

Some low-carb diets let you eat large amounts of foods that are extremely high in saturated fats. That's why the American Heart Association warns that low-carb diets can raise your cholesterol levels and increase your risk of heart disease, stroke, and diabetes. Recent research suggests that low-carb diets may contribute to certain kinds of cancer.

A low-carb diet can also put an enormous strain on your kidneys. Without carbohydrates to use for fuel, your body switches into a metabolic state called ketosis. When you're in ketosis, you get your energy from ketones—a form of carbon that's created from the breakdown of fat. That sounds like exactly what you're looking for, right? Wrong! It's dangerous to your health. The more ketones you have in your system, the harder your kidneys have to work to filter them, and that can lead to kidney failure. If you already have kidney problems, the situation can be dire: A Harvard study published in the *Annals of Internal Medicine* found that low-carb diets can cause a permanent loss of kidney function in people with reduced kidney function.

WHY LOW-CARB DIETS WON'T WORK LONG TERM

Most people don't experience the negative long-term consequences of low-carb diets only because they quit the diets after just a few weeks. I'd hate to see you waste your time, so take a look at the top five reasons people stop following low-carb diets.

1. THEY'RE FAR TOO COMPLEX

How did you fare in algebra back in high school? Adhering to a low-carb diet requires understanding your body's metabolism and calorie breakdowns, choosing the right portion sizes, and dividing up how many grams of protein, carbs, and fats are in every single food you eat. Some of the recipes in these diet books are so complex, they require more cooking skills—and time—than the average person has.

The 5-Factor Diet Difference: With the 5-Factor Diet, the recipes are as tasty as those you'd find in the trendiest Hollywood restaurants, but they're still designed so that anyone—no matter how limited his or her culinary skills—can whip up nutritious meals and snacks with little effort. And as for math, you can count to 5, can't you? Because that's all I'll ever ask you to do.

2. THEY TAKE UP TOO MUCH TIME

Because of their complexity, low-carb diets simply require too much time to think, organize, and implement. That's why many people give up on low-carb diets early on.

The 5-Factor Diet Difference: My clients' time is extremely limited and incredibly valuable. So is yours. I realize that the only way to keep you eating right is to make it easier to eat right. That's why all of the recipes in the 5-Factor Diet take no more than 5 minutes of prep time before cooking.

3. THEY AREN'T VERY SOCIAL

Eating a meal should be a social experience, yet low-carb diets leave many people feeling like the odd man out. You can't enjoy a meal at a restaurant with your friends when you're too busy trying to find a low-carb option on the menu and calculating protein grams. That's why most people end up cheating on these diets when they go out to eat.

The 5-Factor Diet Difference: Most of my celebrity clients work in an industry that practically forces them to be sociable. At the same time, however, privacy is very important to them. Like you, they need a diet program they can use anywhere *without* advertising the fact that they're dieting. The 5-Factor Diet works at home, on the road, or in any restaurant, so you'll never again have to choose between food and friends.

4. THEY DON'T SHOW YOU HOW TO EXERCISE

Low-carb diets may mention how essential exercise is for losing weight, but none of them go into detail about how you should exercise. That's like telling people a road trip will be much faster and smoother if they buy a faster engine, and then never saying where to find one!

The 5-Factor Diet Difference: The 5-Factor Diet is one of the few nutritional programs out there that show you the right way to eat *and* the right way to exercise.

5. THEY SLOW YOU DOWN ON EVERY LEVEL

Your brain relies on carbohydrates to help it function. Yet these low-carb diets reduce the amount of carbs you eat to a trickle of what your brain desperately needs. No wonder low-carb, high-protein dieters tend to have a tough time concentrating. They also end up suffering from fatigue, which leaves them with less energy for exercise.

The 5-Factor Diet Difference: With the 5-Factor Diet, not only will you be free to eat carbohydrates, but you'll also learn which ones are best for your body. And while other diets may shock you when you see what you *can't* eat, with my 5-Factor Diet, you'll be amazed at what you *can* eat.

BEWARE OF THESE POPULAR LOW-CARB DIETS

You've just heard all the negatives that low-carb diets have in common, but each version is also controversial for a variety of its own reasons. Here are the facts you deserve to know.

ATKINS DIET

This popular low-carb diet contends that overconsumption of carbohydrates is the main reason for obesity. Bread, pastas, and potatoes are to be avoided on this plan. Therefore, the Atkins diet severely restricts how many carbohydrates you eat each day and limits your daily calories to between 1,200 and 1,800. The reason this diet is appealing to many people is that you do lose a certain amount of weight—plus you can eat fatty meats, certain fried foods, high-fat dairy products, cheese, eggs, and even butter.

All the freedom the Atkins diet offers comes at a price. Because it's so anti-carb, the diet is lacking in fruits, whole grains, and fiber. Your body misses out on many important nutrients, including vitamin B, vitamin C, and other phytonutrients that boost your immune system. You may drop a few quick pounds by stripping most carbohydrates from your diet, but it's mostly water weight and muscle tissue—and it may place you at risk for a series of short- and long-term health problems.

Your risk of developing osteoporosis may increase because the diet lowers your calcium intake. Research published in the *American Journal of Kidney Disease* found that healthy subjects who tried the Atkins diet experienced calcium losses that were 65 percent greater than normal.

Your risk of heart disease may increase because the diet encourages people to eat fatty meats and certain cheeses, which are high in artery-blocking saturated fats.

Further, according to the National Weight Control Registry, which monitors the diets of more than 2,500 people who have maintained a 30-pound weight loss for at least a year, fewer than 1 percent of these successful dieters use a low-carb, high-protein plan that resembles the Atkins diet.

ZONE DIET

The Zone Diet is a rigid high-protein, low-carb diet. It requires you to divide every single meal you eat using a 40/30/30 ratio: 40 percent carbohydrate, 30 percent protein, and 30 percent fat.

According to the Zone's creator, most people suffer from insulin imbalances that cause them to put on weight. By eating protein, carbs, and fats in the right proportions, you can correct this imbalance and drop the pounds, along with your risk of developing cardiac diseases, diabetes, depression, cancer, and even PMS.

In order to benefit from the diet, you must follow the calculations to the absolute letter. Dividing the components of every meal you eat can be incredibly complicated and takes the enjoyment out of eating, unless you find pleasure in having to pass a math exam each time you want a meal. This plan is too difficult for anyone with a life to manage, or just to put up with for very long.

I'm sure you have friends who swear by the Zone. I will admit that I've seen people get excited when they lose some weight at the start of the plan. But it's the reduction of total daily calories—1,000 to 1,700 calories a day—that's responsible for the weight loss, not the whole 40/30/30 breakdown. A good portion of the weight loss is water and muscle tissue—two things your body can't afford to lose.

The portion sizes of the carbohydrates you're allowed to eat are so small, you'll forget you even ate them in the first place. Your body won't remember the carbs either, and as a result, you'll never achieve satiety. When you quit this diet you'll have better division skills, but don't count on having a leaner, healthier body.

SOUTH BEACH DIET

The South Beach Diet claims to be different from the Atkins diet because it's not completely anti-carbs; instead it encourages you to eat the "right" kinds of carbs.

The first stage of this three-stage diet requires you to stop eating potatoes, pasta, bread, candy, cookies, alcohol, ice cream, baked goods, and sugar. But giving up all of these vices at once is nearly impossible. It's ironic that the South Beach Diet starts off by saying how the Zone Diet is not the answer and the Atkins diet is too severe. Yet once you look at it carefully, you'll realize South Beach is a mix of Atkins and Zone. And the third and final stage is just the daily allowances recommended by the American Dietetic Association.

South Beach also claims that you'll drop 8–13 pounds in its first two-week phase. But just like on the Atkins diet, you're losing water and not fat.

CHAPTER 4

The 5-Factor Diet Does Work

Take a deep breath and relax. I want you to know that you're finally about to embark on a diet plan that—unlike the fad diets I've shown you don't work in the long term—you can use for the rest of your life. The only side effect of the 5-Factor Diet is a healthier, fitter body. The only danger is that you may stop traffic when you walk downtown. If you're ready for those kinds of results, let's get started.

Many celebrity trainers handle only the exercise portion of their clients' fitness programs. I incorporate both exercise and nutritional information. In fact, that's the core of my business as I work with thousands of people face-to-face, over the phone, and online. I work with people who live all over the world, from South America and Europe to North America, Asia, and Australia. That global perspective has shown me that people eat badly all over the world. I had to create a diet plan that would address the fitness and nutritional needs of anyone, no matter where he or she is from or what his or her nutrition habits and culture.

THE 5-FACTOR DIET IS BASED ON WELL-ESTABLISHED SCIENCE

Most fad diets will base their entire eating plan on one study; other diets take one specific scientific finding and spin an entire eating plan around it. That's not very balanced, is it? Those kinds of programs can never deliver the realistic, healthy diet you need.

The 5-Factor Diet is different. Its components are based on well-established science and on many sound, time-honored studies. These aren't studies that will be refuted six months after this book is published. The 5-Factor Diet and 5-Factor Recipes are supported by unchallenged and rock-solid research that has existed for years—in some cases, the studies were done long before I worked with my first client. (See "5-Factor Golden Rules," page 41, for more on the science behind this diet.) And the 5-Factor Diet is easy to follow: Anyone can use it and see results—no matter who you are or where you're from.

YOU'LL LEARN TO LOVE THE NUMBER 5

The 5-Factor Diet starts and ends with the number 5. In fact, everything in the 5-Factor Diet revolves around the number 5. Here's how my menu plan breaks down—in 5s, of course—to help you stay on track.

5 IS THE NUMBER OF MEALS YOU'LL EAT EVERY DAY

There is no skipping meals on the 5-Factor Diet—and with recipes as tasty as the ones I have developed for you, you won't want to pass up a single bite. Each day, you'll eat your typical three meals (breakfast, lunch, and dinner) plus two healthy snacks, one in midmorning and one in midafternoon.

To figure out when you should eat, start by adding up how many hours you're awake during the day—from the time you get out of bed until you turn out the light at night—and divide that number by 5. The resulting number is roughly the number of hours I want you to wait between meals. For example, if you get up at 7 a.m. and go to bed at 11 p.m., you're awake for 16 hours. Divide 16 by 5 and you get a little over three hours, so you should eat at 8 a.m., 11 a.m., 2 p.m., 5 p.m., and 8 p.m.

As you can already imagine, eating 5 meals a day ensures that you'll never feel hungry or deprived. (In "5 Meals a Day Are Key," page 35, I'll get into more detail about the science behind why eating 5 meals is vital to seeing the best results.)

5 IS HOW MANY ELEMENTS EACH MEAL SHOULD INCLUDE

That may sound daunting, but it's easier than it sounds. There are no particular foods I want you to eat. Rather, I want you to make sure every meal or snack you eat is a mix of five elements: protein, low- to moderate-glycemic carbohydrates, healthy fats, and fiber, along with a sugar-free beverage to wash it down. This is the heart of the 5-Factor Diet.

I'll go into more detail soon, but for now just know that *you* get to decide what foods to eat from these five categories. All I ask is that you incorporate all five on your plate at every meal. To make it effortless, the recipes in this book (see "5-Factor Recipes," page 110) all meet the 5-Factor criteria. If you follow my menu, it'll be easy to stick to the 5-Factor Diet.

5 IS THE MAXIMUM NUMBER OF STEPS, MINUTES, AND MAIN INGREDIENTS EACH RECIPE REQUIRES

I know one of the hardest things about dieting is learning how to prepare what's healthy. With my 5-Factor Diet, I've removed that problem from the equation. Every one of my recipes uses 5 or fewer core ingredients, requires 5 steps or fewer to prepare, and takes only 5 minutes to prepare (not counting cook time). Now you'll always have time to watch what you eat.

Ben Foster ACTOR, STAR IN THE MOVIE *X-MEN: THE LAST STAND*

"Harley Pasternak has developed an extraordinary program for health and fitness. No trends, no gimmicks. Only serious results. It's user friendly, and it is the most effective way to ensure long-term health."

5 IS HOW MANY DAYS A WEEK YOU SHOULD EXERCISE

Exercise is the important factor that most diets gloss over, yet it's critical in the battle to lose weight and make your body healthy, strong, and more injury resistant. I said this in my first book, *5-Factor Fitness*: Eating is 50 percent of the getting-fit equation, and exercise is the other 50 percent.

To get the full benefit of the 5-Factor Diet, you must exercise. That's why I've included a "New 5-Factor Hollywood Workout" (see page 82) with the 5-Factor Diet. It makes it easy to exercise five days a week, so you will always feel great while maximizing your progress.

5 IS THE NUMBER OF FOOD TYPES YOU'LL STOCK IN YOUR KITCHEN

As part of the 5-Factor Diet, I have determined the 5 types of foods—proteins, carbohydrates, condiments, snacks, and beverages—that you should always have on hand. I've further broken this down into the 5-Factor Must-Have Foods, comprising are five of the best nutritional picks from each category, for 25 essential foods you'll always want to have on hand. (For details, see "5-Factor Must-Have Foods," page 50.) There's no guesswork with my eating plan.

WHY THE 5-FACTOR DIET WILL WORK FOR YOU

I call my plan the 5-Factor Diet, but truth be told, it's not as much a diet as a lifestyle. It works for a number of reasons, all of which should resonate with you, especially if you've ever failed at dieting in the past. It works because I can make the following five important promises to you.

1. YOU'LL NEVER FEEL HUNGRY OR DEPRIVED

Have you ever been on a diet that gives you a feeling of emptiness in your stomach, as if you haven't eaten for weeks? That sensation simply doesn't exist on my 5-Factor Diet for several reasons. One of the main principles behind the 5-Factor Diet is eating 5 times a day. It's hard to be hungry with 5 meals a day!

Eating 5 meals spaced evenly throughout the day also keeps your blood sugar (also called blood glucose) stable, which naturally keeps your appetite in check. I've found that eating frequent meals has an important effect on eating habits. My clients tell me that they always feel as if they're either just about to eat, eating, or just finishing a meal. That's good because it means they never feel desperate for food.

Another reason you won't feel hungry is that you'll combine five very important things—protein, low- or moderate-glycemic carbs, fiber, healthy fats, and a sugar-free beverage—in every meal. (See "The Ideal 5-Factor Meal," page 42, for more details.) These five foods work with one another not just to improve your health and help you lose weight but also to leave you feeling fuller.

Never feeling hungry or deprived is exactly the condition I want for you, because that will keep you from eating more than you should. In

---

MY 5-FACTOR DIET PROMISES

1. You'll never feel hungry or deprived.

2. You'll enjoy a "cheat" day every week.

3. You don't have to buy supplements.

4. You won't spend hours in the kitchen.

5. You can use the 5-Factor Diet everywhere you go.

---

studies, critical hospital patients who were given the option to administer their own morphine for pain actually chose to use less than what their doctors would have given them. Similarly, you may find you eat less on the 5-Factor Diet simply because it puts *you* in control—instead of dictating exactly what you can and can't have.

The 5-Factor Diet isn't based on restrictions. You won't be cutting carbs or eliminating sugar or any entire food group. In fact, half of this book is filled with recipes for delicious pizza, spaghetti, pancakes, burritos, and many other dishes that most people crave. And it's easy to fit the foods you like into the 5-Factor Diet even if you don't follow my recipes all the time.

2. YOU'LL ENJOY A "CHEAT" DAY EVERY SINGLE WEEK

On the 5-Factor Diet, you're rewarded each week with the chance to eat whatever you want—guilt free. Why would any diet allow you to do such a thing?

You must remember this: Living healthfully should not come at the expense of living well. I think it's awfully sad when somebody refuses to eat her own birthday cake. Or when someone visits the most delicious French restaurant in New York City but orders only a green salad because he's dieting. I would ask those people, "Why are you alive? What good is your health if you aren't enjoying life?" The 5-Factor program never forgets that.

Common GRAMMY NOMINATED MUSICIAN, ACTOR

"Being trained by Harley has made me realize that physical fitness is part of the spirit, body, and mind connection. His insight and energy toward training and health have been a blessing toward improving my life."

Everyone needs a mini meal vacation, if you will. Taking off one day a week is a catharsis. It's a mental relief. It re-empowers you, so you never feel like you're in a diet prison. In fact, an occasional high-calorie day may be just what your body needs to lose weight. Researchers at the National Institutes of Health discovered that subjects who for one day ate twice as many calories as they do normally increased their metabolism by 9 percent in the 24 hours that followed. So cheating one day can help you burn calories—as long as you return to the plan the next day.

If you're worried that cheating may make you want to stray the next day as well, don't fret. Most likely, the cheat day is exactly what you need to prove how well the 5-Factor Diet is working.

It's a lot like using premium fuel in your car. You don't realize how well your car runs on it until the day you decide to save a dime and pour in a few gallons of cheap fuel instead. Suddenly your car sputters and the motor doesn't seem to respond as well. It'll be the same for you when you put away the premium 5-Factor Recipes and fill up on junk.

That's one of the advantages to a cheat day. I want you to cheat so you can see how sluggish you feel when you slip back into old habits. I guarantee that after a few cheats, you'll begin to ask yourself afterward, "Was that really worth it?" You may find yourself craving pizza all week and then, after you have it, realize the main reason you craved it was because you weren't allowed to have it. I can tell you that after my cheat day, I feel mentally and physically different in a way that reminds me how much healthier my body feels when I follow the 5-Factor Diet.

You can pick any one day of the week to splurge, but I suggest you try to make it the same day each week so you always have something to look forward to. Of course, if you know there's a day in the week that's going to be more of a challenge foodwise—perhaps you've been invited to a party or you have a work dinner—then feel free to switch days.

Personally, I prefer Sunday for my cheat day because it's usually a day that's more social, and a day when I'm more likely to be around the sinful foods I've been dodging diligently all week. For me, Sunday also feels like the official end of the week. By making their cheat day Sunday, many of my clients feel as if they are building up to something that they earn through sticking to the plan.

3. YOU DON'T NEED SUPPLEMENTS

It strikes me as odd that so many people are willing to shell out large amounts of money for flavorless pill and powder supplements to add nutrients to their diets—nutrients they could be getting simply by eating the right combination of foods. Those foods would also fill them up so they wouldn't binge on the nutritionless fare that was causing them to be nutrient deprived in the first place.

While writing this book, I looked up the word *supplement* in the dictionary. By definition, it's "something added to make up for a deficiency." If you're eating the right foods according to the 5-Factor Diet, you never have to worry about being deficient in any nutritional area, and you never have to spend a dime on supplements. The 5-Factor Diet is based on the inherent nutritional value of real foods. It is designed to give you the right amount of macro- and micronutrients that your body needs—nutrients you may not be getting from your diet right now. (If you have an allergy or a religious obligation that prevents you from eating a particular food—such as eggs, milk, or shellfish—the 5-Factor Diet offers plenty of other options that are equally abundant in nutrients. That way, you can tailor the diet to accommodate your needs without missing out on nutrition.)

Is it OK to take a multivitamin while on the 5-Factor Diet? Of course it is. In fact, I encourage you to take multivitamins, but not because the 5-Factor Diet is deficient. Certain foods—especially fruits, vegetables, and

> "I'm a baseball player with the Los Angeles Dodgers, and the 5-Factor program has changed my life. I ended up losing 40 pounds before spring training, and the level of fitness that I have achieved has helped me have the best season of my career. 5-Factor has become my off-season and in-season training program. Thanks, Harley!"
>
> **Casey Hoorelbeke** WEIGHT LOST SO FAR: **40 lbs.**

meats—can lose a percentage of their vitamins and minerals, depending on how they're prepared or when they're picked. A multivitamin serves as backup insurance for your body, just in case some of your foods have reduced levels of micro- and macronutrients.

Most people can choose a regular over-the-counter multivitamin from the drugstore. However, women who are no longer menstruating, as well as men, should choose types that don't contain iron.

There are a few supplements that can make life easier because of their convenience. For example, if you simply can't get your hands on another protein source to include in a meal, I encourage you to use protein powders and high-protein RTD (Ready to Drink) meal replacement drinks. In fact, I put RTDs on my list of "5-Factor Must-Have Foods" (page 61).

4. YOU WON'T SPEND HOURS IN THE KITCHEN

Who has time to bake a casserole? I don't, my clients don't, and I'm sure you don't either. Whether you're the head of a corporation or the head of your household, time is tight for everyone. Lack of time is a big reason why a lot of us eat badly to begin with. It often seems far easier and faster to swing by a drive-through or grab a packaged snack than it is to prepare a healthy dish from scratch.

It's a myth that cooking healthy has to take lots of time. To prove that fact, I designed all the 5-Factor Recipes in this book to be prepared in five minutes or less. How is that possible? Every recipe has a maximum of 5 key ingredients. Each recipe has 5 or fewer steps to follow. With the 5-Factor Diet, you can stop watching the clock and start watching your shrinking waistline.

Even if you decide to create your own tasty dishes in addition to mine, you'll see how every food I've recommended for you to eat is easy to prepare. And because you don't count calories or portion sizes with the 5-Factor Diet, you don't waste time worrying about anything but enjoying your food.

5. YOU CAN USE THE 5-FACTOR DIET EVERYWHERE

Some of my clients are musicians, and when they're on tour they can be in a different city every night. So I needed to create a nutritional plan that they could stick to no matter where they landed the next day. That's perhaps the greatest gift the 5-Factor Diet offers anyone who wants to lose weight: It makes it easy to take your healthy habits with you outside your home and wherever you go.

The 5-Factor Diet doesn't require that you eat certain foods or certain portions. There are no strange supplements to order, no meetings to attend, no refrigerators filled with packaged meals. All you have to do in order to stick to this plan is eat five meals a day, with each meal containing a protein, a low- or moderate-glycemic carbohydrate, fiber, a healthy fat, and a sugar-free beverage.

With so few guidelines, you can see that it's easy to do the 5-Factor Diet anywhere. You can go to Jamaica and have jerk chicken with rice and peas and be eating the 5-Factor Diet. You can head to Spain and have brown rice with seafood. You can take the 5-Factor Diet with you as your own personal travel partner—anywhere in the world—and get results!

5 Meals a Day Are Key

Research has shown that eating five meals a day rather than the traditional three (or two, for those who unwisely skip breakfast) is optimal for maintaining healthy and stable insulin levels.

When I attended the University of Toronto years ago, my professors included Dr. David Jenkins and Dr. Thomas M. S. Wolever. Those names may not mean anything to you—and if they do, then I'm proud of you—but they did to me. You see, Jenkins and Wolever were two of the world's leading active glycemic index (GI) researchers. In fact, it was they who created the glycemic index—the system that measures, on a scale of 0 to 100, the body's blood sugar response to carbohydrates. They also suggested eating smaller meals throughout the day—"grazing" instead of gorging. A few years after that research was published, I was lucky, and honored, to study under both of them. They have had a profound

> "I wanted to lose my belly, but I was completely unmotivated to work out because most programs looked too long and complicated to start. I found 5-Factor to be well structured and extremely easy to maintain. In just eight weeks, I lost approximately 16 pounds and have managed to keep it off!"
>
> **Yvon Brunet** AGE: **48** WEIGHT LOST SO FAR: **16 lbs.**

influence on me, both personally and professionally. They're the reason you're holding this book.

WHY 5 MEALS A DAY WORKS

It started the day I decided to put my professors' theories to the test. At first I tried eating six meals a day, but I found it didn't feel very natural because I was used to eating breakfast, lunch, and dinner. Trying to squeeze in six meals felt like I was stuffing myself. Five meals is a lot easier and more sensible to maintain. I had my regular breakfast, lunch, and dinner and added snacks in between. As soon as I stuck with 5 meals, I felt—and saw—the results. From there, I researched ways of making my 5 meals even more effective at fighting fat, building muscle, and improving my overall health. The result is the 5-Factor Diet.

By following this 5-meal-a-day plan, you are changing the way you eat and the reasons why you are eating. If you eat on a schedule, rather than waiting until you're hungry and *must* eat, you become proactive with your diet instead of reactive. *You* are in control of what—and how much—you consume. Once you're in that driver's seat, you get to control how your body looks, feels, and performs.

5-FACTOR DIET BENEFITS

When you stick to my 5-meal-a-day 5-Factor Diet, you'll benefit from five important changes to your body that most diets simply can't offer.

1. IT LOWERS YOUR INSULIN LEVELS

Eating 5 meals a day—and eating the right combinations of foods—can prevent your body from releasing excess insulin into its system. By eating 5 normal-size meals instead of the usual two or three big meals, you tend to eat less food at each meal. Eating less food at each meal means you naturally end up eating less sugar. As a result, less insulin is released and you store less fat.

Keeping your insulin levels low all day long isn't important just for losing fat. It's also necessary if you want to avoid the dangerous medical condition hyperinsulinemia, which occurs when you have too much insulin in your blood too often. This condition is harmful to your long-term health. It also affects you daily by lowering your concentration, diminishing your memory, and causing headaches and dizziness. Sticking with the 5-meals-a-day rule of the 5-Factor Diet prevents all of the above problems, so all you have to do is eat instead of worry.

2. IT GIVES YOU MORE ENERGY ALL DAY

Despite all the other health benefits of the 5-Factor Diet, my guess is that your main goal is to lose weight. Following my system certainly will make that happen. But what really gives you an edge over other dieters is the enormous amount of energy you'll have on this plan. Eating 5 smaller meals a day keeps a nice, steady stream of calories flowing, so you feel more energized and less sluggish. Eating larger meals less often has the exact opposite effect—Thanksgiving, anyone?

You also get an energy boost on the 5-Factor Diet because you're eating protein at all 5 meals. Here's why: One of protein's most important amino acids is tyrosine, which can increase your mental alertness and energy by elevating the brain chemicals dopamine and norepinephrine. By eating protein 5 times a day as opposed to two or three times a day, you release these chemicals twice as often for extra energy all day. That's a nutritional secret many fad dieters—and even the general population, for the most part—never take advantage of. How many times have you seen someone snack on pretzels, fruits, or other carbohydrates without eating anything else with it? When it comes to staying energized, that's a big no-no.

What you decide to do with your newfound energy is up to you. Maybe you'll use it to exercise more effectively. Or maybe you'll use that extra burst to get more done at work or focus on a relationship. Whatever you do, I promise you'll have energy when you need it—always.

3. IT IGNITES YOUR METABOLISM

Did you know that you burn more calories eating than when you're at rest? It's ironic but true. Every time you eat, your body uses up a certain amount of energy—and calories—digesting, absorbing, metabolizing, and storing your meal. In fact, about 5 to 15 percent of your total calories is spent on digestion alone. It's called the "thermic effect of food" (TEF): The more often you eat, the more often your metabolism revs up as your body processes the food. That's yet another scientific reason why there are five meals spaced throughout the day in the 5-Factor Diet.

I like to think of the metabolism as a pinwheel—you know, the toy that looks like a mini fan on a stick that spins when you blow air through it. Your metabolism is like a pinwheel, and you want to keep it spinning. The faster and longer you can make it spin, the more calories you burn.

Each time you eat a meal, it's like blowing air on a pinwheel. If you wait too long before blowing again, the pinwheel starts to slow down. To keep your metabolism constantly spinning, you must time your meals so that just as your body begins to slow down, more food arrives to revive it. Eating 5 meals a day keeps these breezes flowing and your metabolism spinning.

> **5-FACTOR DIET BENEFITS**
> 1. It lowers your insulin levels.
> 2. It gives you more energy all day.
> 3. It ignites your metabolism.
> 4. It improves your mood.
> 5. It reduces stress.

My diet gives you even more of a TEF advantage because of the foods you eat at each meal. Protein has a TEF roughly twice as high as that of carbohydrates and fat. That's why simply raising the amount of protein you eat daily from 15 percent of your total calories (the amount most people eat) to 35 percent (the amount I want you to eat) will increase your TEF by 21 calories daily. That number may seem tiny, but remember, the effect is cumulative.

4. IT IMPROVES YOUR MOOD

Have you ever felt agitated, depressed, or irritable during the day, but you couldn't pinpoint what was causing it? It might be from eating less often than you should—something eating 5 meals a day can fix.

John Mayer GRAMMY-WINNING SINGER AND SONGWRITER

"5-Factor is not a diet, in the sense that there's nothing to fall off of. There's nothing to say good-bye to, and nothing to long for. It is almost too good to be true!"

I've explained that eating less often and having bigger meals raises your insulin levels so you end up storing excess calories as fat. There's also an emotional downside to this situation. When you eat less often and have larger meals, your body not only releases insulin but also overcompensates by releasing too much insulin, just to be sure it's doing its job. The result is that your body removes more blood sugar than necessary, causing a net deficit in your body's supply of glucose. Having less energy leaves you feeling less happy and more miserable, no matter how happy you normally are. Eating 5 smaller meals a day can prevent this and improve your mood—unless you have a good reason to be angry or upset!

On the 5-Factor Diet, you're also protecting yourself from mood swings by eating a low- to moderate-glycemic carbohydrate at every meal. Research performed at the Massachusetts Institute of Technology found that eating less than 50 grams of carbohydrates daily can cause a significant drop in the chemical serotonin, which your brain releases to help regulate mood and appetite.

When your serotonin level dips, you're more susceptible to feeling depressed and anxious. Getting enough serotonin on a regular basis raises how much of the chemical your body produces. Eating 5 meals a day—with carbs at each meal—keeps your levels steady so you never encounter the kind of emotional highs and lows you may have felt on other diets.

The 5-Factor Diet and 5-Factor Recipes also incorporate plenty of foods that are rich in folate—a mineral that helps lower homocysteine, an amino acid that's been shown to cause depression at high levels—as well as healthy fats and essential fatty acids, which have been shown to help naturally treat depression.

5. IT REDUCES STRESS

Eating is important for a reason most people don't quite understand: It's a time to relax and put your life on pause for a moment. A meal is a time for reflection for many people—or at least it should be. It's a time to rest and think.

I want you to look at each meal as "your" time. No matter how stressful your day is, or how angry your boss is making you, I want you to use your five mealtimes to simply pause and ponder, even if it's only for a few minutes. Taking a break isn't just healthy for your mind; it's also beneficial to your body. Taking the time to make a meal, then sit down and eat it, forces you to do something that you might not do otherwise during the day.

As a workaholic, I made a New Year's resolution a few years ago to find a balance in life. I wanted to speak to my parents more often. I wanted to read more. I wanted to spend more time focusing on me instead of all the work that was always piling up around me.

I used my 5 meals a day as a no-excuse way to live up to that promise. They gave me five opportunities in the day to reach out and say hello to my mother or read a chapter in a book. They helped bring balance to my day. I felt calmer and less stressed by the time each meal was over.

Studies have shown that the more stressful your life is, the higher your odds of being overweight. A study performed at the New York Academy of Sciences found that most women who face chronic stress suffer from a condition called stress overeating, caused by the hormone cortisol, which your body releases when under stress. Not only is cortisol toxic to your immune system, but it stimulates appetite, which may be why the study's subjects overate during stressful times.

A study from Yale University found that women dealing with stress typically may develop excess fat around their waistlines and surrounding their organs. The study theorized that there are more cortisol-sensitive receptors within fat cells in your belly than any other areas of your body. That means stressing out about your belly could keep you from losing it—if you don't find the time to unwind, that is.

Exercising regularly and adhering to a healthy diet can lower your stress and help keep your cortisol levels low. Of course, those are both things you'll be doing naturally when you follow my 5-Factor Diet. Taking the time to reflect with each meal can help curb your daily stress even further, helping you keep off the fat.

CHAPTER 6

5-Factor Golden Rules

When I was a graduate student doing nutrition research for Canada's Department of National Defense, I learned all about the biochemistry of food and its effects on the body. What always amazed me was that amid all the science, there were 5 clear-as-day factors that were universally ideal for losing weight, maintaining lean muscle, and improving overall health. It is these 5 rules that became the scientific basis for my 5-Factor Diet.

THE SCIENCE BEHIND THE 5-FACTOR DIET

Scientific factor #1. Protein is the building block of the most important parts of our bodies, from muscles, hormones, and enzymes to skin, organs, and blood.

Scientific factor #2. All carbohydrates are not created equal, as proven by the glycemic index, which is the system that measures on a scale of 0 to 100 the body's blood sugar response to carbohydrates. It's healthier to avoid foods ranked high on the glycemic index and eat low-glycemic carbohydrates instead.

Scientific factor #3. Fiber is vital to the body, as proven by overwhelming research: It has the power to lower everything from bad cholesterol and blood pressure to the risk of certain types of cancers. It also helps keep your digestive system regular.

Scientific factor #4. Not all fats are evil. In fact, healthy fats are an important part of a good diet. Studies show that our hormones, nerves, reproductive system, skin, and hundreds of other parts of the body rely on fat to function properly—yet our society desperately tries to remove every last bit of fat from our foods.

Scientific fact #5. Water is essential to life. Unfortunately, many people use thirst as an excuse to consume sugar and excessive calories.

Using these scientific and nutritional facts, I created the 5-Factor Diet, which—unlike fad diets—is guaranteed to stand the test of time.

THE IDEAL 5-FACTOR MEAL

My diet works because it combines the right 5 types of foods—protein, carbohydrates, fiber, healthy fats, and beverages—in each meal. Each of these 5 Factors is critical to your nutritional success. It's simple: At every meal eat one food from each of the five categories. It's a program that's nutritionally sound and easy to use for the rest of your life.

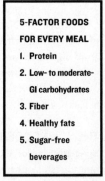

5-FACTOR FOODS FOR EVERY MEAL
1. Protein
2. Low- to moderate-GI carbohydrates
3. Fiber
4. Healthy fats
5. Sugar-free beverages

Think of every 5-Factor Diet meal as a shopping trip to a five-story department store, which you can't leave until you've purchased something from all five floors. That's the simplicity of the 5-Factor Diet, only instead of a store, it's your plate. Instead of having to buy something from every floor, you must eat something from the five 5-Factor food categories.

It's the easiest and simplest way to move toward a leaner, healthier body. Here is a closer look at each food category, with all the details on why it's important and information on proper portion size.

1. PROTEIN

Every meal or snack should contain a low-fat protein such as chicken breast, fish, seafood, egg whites, or cottage cheese. Aim for one-third of your total calories to come from protein, which is vital for maintaining muscle tissue and regulating metabolism.

Protein is No. 1 on this list for several good reasons. First, it helps you feel fuller longer. In recent studies, subjects who ate high-protein, moderate-carbohydrate meals (which is exactly what's recommended in the 5-Factor Diet and the breakdown of every 5-Factor Recipe you'll find in this book) had a greater feeling of fullness after meals that lasted longer during the day than did subjects who ate high-fat meals. That's because there's a certain amount of fat found in animal-based protein like chicken or fish. That may sound like a step in the wrong direction if you want to lose fat, but staying fuller for a longer period of time can curb your hunger in between meals.

EAT THE 5-FACTOR DIET ANYWHERE!

You don't have to stray from the 5-Factor Diet when dining out. Here are a few of my favorite combinations to order at different-style restaurants.

IF YOU'RE DINING ...	ORDER ...
American	Turkey burger
Canadian	Grilled ostrich and a bowl of lentil soup
Chinese	Black bean and shrimp stir-fry
Cuban	Fish soup or grilled chicken with black beans
Greek	Chicken shish kabob or Greek salad
Indian	Tandoori chicken with basmati rice
Italian	Branzino, minestrone soup, or tomato-basil salad
Jamaican	Jerk chicken breasts or rice and beans
Japanese	Seaweed salad, miso soup, sashimi, or teriyaki chicken
Mexican	Chicken fajitas

Because protein helps you maintain muscle, it also helps raise your resting metabolism. It takes more calories to maintain muscle than fat, so the more muscle you have, the more calories you burn throughout the day. Eating plenty of protein and following the 5-Factor Hollywood Workout will help you build more muscle, thus revving up your metabolism.

The best perk about protein is that out of the three macronutrients—protein, carbohydrates, and fat—it's the most difficult to store as body fat. When you eat more fat than your body needs, your body stores it as fat. When you eat more simple carbohydrates than your body needs, blood sugar levels spike. This causes your body to release excess insulin, which helps speed up the conversions of carb calories into fat.

However, when you eat more protein, your body doesn't require as much insulin to metabolize it. Having less insulin in your system lowers your odds of having any excess calories converted to fat. Plus your body has to convert the protein into carbohydrates before it can be converted into fat. All that takes a lot of work, which is why most excess protein leaves the body before it has a chance to become an extra pant size.

The one type of protein I don't recommend is nuts. Some nutritionists sing their praises because they are low in carbohydrates, but most nuts, in general, receive greater than three-fourths of their calories from fat. Although nuts are often considered a major protein source, in truth many of them contain only small amounts of low-quality protein that is incomplete (lacking one or more essential amino acids) or is not bio-available (that is, the body can't use it).

Instead of nuts, pick lower-fat, more-complete protein sources such as egg whites, fish, lean beef, chicken breast, turkey breast, and fat-free milk. You'll maximize your intake of quality protein while minimizing your intake of bad fats.

2. CARBOHYDRATES

Every meal should contain a carbohydrate that ranks low or moderate on the glycemic index. Good choices include vegetables, wild rice, beans, lentils, oatmeal, sweet potato, and quinoa.

Carbohydrates have taken a lot of flak lately, thanks to poorly conceived fad diets. The truth is that carbs are responsible for fueling your body and providing most of the energy you need to live. That's why every meal

> "I had always been interested in fitness, but it wasn't until reading your book that I finally corrected all my mistakes. I was overloading on carbohydrates, eating three meals a day, and didn't know the right balance of protein and carbs. Thanks to 5-Factor, I learned about eating the right types of foods and the benefits of having 5 small meals a day."
>
> **Michael Bigman** WEIGHT LOST SO FAR: **8 lbs.**

you eat should have at least two portions (that's 50 percent of your total calories) of some type of low- to moderate-glycemic carbohydrate.

Why am I not anti-carb like other nutrition experts? Because eating a mixture of fibrous carbohydrates and protein keeps you sharp. You see, carbohydrates are absorbed into the system much faster than protein is, so eating a mixture of protein and the right carbs increases your alertness by burning calories at staggered times. That gives you a feeling of satiety and an even release of energy throughout the day. That's energy your body can use to exercise later on. Carbs also help the fat in your diet be more efficiently metabolized. Basically, fat burns in a carbohydrate flame. Most low-GI carbohydrates also contain some soluble fiber (see "Fiber," page 46), which is also important.

I've mentioned the glycemic index (GI), which is a system that rates carbohydrate foods based on how quickly your body converts them into glucose. Foods that break down rapidly—such as starchy foods—release glucose quickly into your blood and rank higher on the index. Foods that break down slowly—such as spinach and cabbage—slowly release glucose into your blood, so they rank lower on the index.

The problem with high-glycemic food is that when its sugar enters your blood, your pancreas immediately has to produce insulin to help regulate it. Your body's natural response to extra insulin in your system is to store whatever calories it can find—whether from carbs, protein, or fat—as unwanted body fat.

Low- to moderate-glycemic carbs release glucose at a much slower pace, so your pancreas produces less insulin. Less insulin means less body fat—need I say more? That's what makes low- to moderate-glycemic foods such a critical part of the 5-Factor Diet.

Try to choose carbs with a glycemic level under 80. These foods can give your body enough all-day energy without causing an insulin surge that may store excess body fat. I prefer fruits and vegetables because they're nutrient rich, low in calories, and water based, which means they're packed with water that fills your stomach. Good picks that are low to moderate on the GI scale include apples, black beans, broccoli, cabbage, carrots, celery, cherries, chickpeas, cucumbers, grapefruits, green peas, lentils, lettuce, lima beans, mushrooms, onions, pears, peaches, peppers, plums, oatmeal, oranges, snow peas, spinach, strawberries, sweet potatoes, and wild rice.

3. FIBER

Every meal should contain 5 to 10 grams of fiber. The health benefits of fiber are numerous: It reduces your risk of developing diabetes and some cancers and lowers your overall blood cholesterol. Fiber slows down the release of glucose (again, the substance your body uses for energy) into the bloodstream, preventing your body from burning through its energy stores too quickly. Fiber even increases how quickly your meals pass into your stomach. The faster you can move food through your digestive system, the less fat and calories you'll absorb. But most important, fiber leaves you feeling full, so you end up eating less at every meal.

Fiber comes in two forms: soluble and insoluble. Both are valuable assets, though, for entirely different reasons. Soluble fiber—found in foods such as peas, oat bran, seeds, beans, barley, lentils, and apples—is digestible and helps lower your risk of developing heart disease and high cholesterol. Insoluble fiber—found in wheat bran, whole grains, vegetables, and beans—is not digested or absorbed by your body but passes through instead, which helps improve the health of your digestive system and colon. Insoluble fiber can also help you drop a few extra pounds. A USDA study found that eating 36 grams of fiber each day can prevent your body from absorbing 130 calories a day.

Kanye West SINGER/SONGWRITER

"The 5-Factor Diet saved me on tour. I can't believe there is healthy food that tastes this good. I've never been in better shape!"

You should eat at least 20 to 30 grams of fiber each day. You can have even more than that—if you can handle it—but do make sure you're getting at least the bare minimum by eating 5 grams at each meal. Over your five meals, you'll ensure you're getting at least 25 grams daily. Ideally, I'd like you to eat 10 grams of fiber at breakfast, lunch, and dinner and 5 grams per snack, which would place you right around 40 grams of fiber a day.

That might sound like a lot, but simply throwing a few handfuls of fiber-rich beans (about ½ cup) into a meal adds around 8 grams of fiber. Some of my favorite fiber-rich foods include whole-grain cereal, brown or wild rice, beans and lentils, no-flour wheat breads, and whole veggies and fruits that have edible skins or seeds.

4. HEALTHY FATS

If your meal contains any fat, it should always be a healthy one—either monounsaturated or polyunsaturated. If you believe it's better to avoid eating fats altogether, think again. Your body needs it—even if your No. 1 mission is to lose body fat. Fat is a major source of energy and helps the body absorb vitamins A, D, E, and K. It also provides taste and consistency, and it helps you feel full so you eat less. Research has even shown that having too little fat in the diet can cause clinical depression. That's because to function properly, your brain needs a certain amount of fat, especially the kind containing omega-3 and omega-6 fatty acids.

Besides, I really don't need to remind you to eat fat because it's almost impossible to avoid. But when you're going to eat a food that contains fat or is cooked in fat, you should stick to the healthy kind—or "good fats," as nutritionists like to call them.

GOOD FATS/BAD FATS: SIMPLE SUBSTITUTIONS

Replacing bad fats with good fats doesn't have to be difficult. Here are five ways to do it that your taste buds won't notice but your body will appreciate.

1. Switch your cooking oil to grapeseed, canola, or extra-virgin olive oil. All three work well under extreme heat.

2. Toss a tiny amount of flaxseed meal on your veggies instead of butter or margarine.

3. If a recipe calls for vegetable shortening, substitute half as much virgin olive oil and a dash of salt.

4. Skip packaged snacks like potato chips and eat seeds instead.

5. Instead of using butter or margarine on your food, try extra-virgin olive oil or flaxseed oil mixed with a dash of salt.

Good fats. Monounsaturated fats are good fats because they don't increase your total cholesterol. In fact, they lower your LDL (bad cholesterol) while simultaneously increasing your HDL (good cholesterol). Monounsaturated fats are found in foods such as fish oil, peanut oil, olive oil, and canola oil.

Polyunsaturated fats have the same positive effect, and they're found in a variety of foods, such as fattier fish like mackerel, albacore tuna, rainbow trout, herring, salmon, and sardines, as well as sunflower oil, canola oil, and flaxseed.

Both monounsaturated and polyunsaturated fats may be "healthy," but they are still fat, and eaten in abundance, they will make you fat. To avoid that, limit your fats to 65 grams a day (or 100 grams maximum).

Bad fats. Saturated fats raise your total blood cholesterol and LDL (bad cholesterol). These fats are hard to avoid; if you can't avoid them, eat them sparingly. Saturated fats are found mostly in animal products such as meat, poultry skin, whole milk, butter, milk chocolate, and egg yolks, as well as in coconut oil, palm oil, and palm kernel oil.

Trans fats, or hydrogenated fats, have the same bad effect on your cholesterol. These are synthetic fats created to give a long shelf life to certain foods. You'll find them in processed foods, commercially prepared baked goods, stick butter, margarine, vegetable shortening, and every bad food you've ever seen made with the last two—including french fries and microwave popcorn. I want you to eliminate trans fats from your diet.

5. SUGAR-FREE BEVERAGES

Every meal should be accompanied by a sugar-free beverage such as water, sugar-free soda, tea, coffee, or an unsweetened energy drink. Your goal is to drink 8 to 12 ounces of a healthy beverage with every meal and snack.

Hydration is important for several reasons. First, for every ounce of excess liquid you drink with your meal, that's one ounce of real estate you steal away from food. More liquid in your belly leaves you feeling fuller and lessens your appetite for your next meal—and throughout the day.

Second, you'll burn more calories all day long. Most people are dehydrated and don't even know it. That's because by the time your thirst mechanism kicks in, your body has already lost about 4 to 5 percent of its water. This condition—called chronic mild dehydration—can affect every biochemical function in your body, including digestion. When your body is well hydrated, it can digest your food with less effort, so even less of it gets stored as body fat. Keeping your digestive system running well also helps it absorb more nutrients as it processes your food.

Third, being properly hydrated may prevent you from eating as much during your next meal or snack. Often people eat because they think they're hungry when they are actually thirsty. That's because thirst triggers the same physical responses as hunger. The next time you feel the urge to eat, try satisfying that urge with a sugar-free beverage instead.

Drinking 8 to 12 ounces at each of your 5 meals guarantees that you'll drink between 40 and 60 ounces a day. But it's not enough to only drink at meals. I recommend that you drink a total of 10 to 12 glasses (roughly 96 ounces), spread throughout the day. If drinking straight water doesn't sound enticing, mix in a very small amount of fruit juice for flavor. Also opt for ice-cold water when possible. Ice-cold water forces your body to burn calories to heat the water up to your body temperature. The effect may be slight, but every little bit helps!

CHAPTER 7

5-Factor
Must-Have
Foods

Although my 5-Factor Diet neither prohibits nor advocates any one food or food group, I have scouted out foods that are ideally suited to the 5-Factor Diet. These foods will keep your diet varied, wholesome, and delicious. I call them the 5-Factor Must-Have Foods. If you keep your fridge and pantry stocked with at least a week's worth of these foods, you'll find that following the 5-Factor Diet is easy and convenient.

There are 5 categories of foods you should always have at the ready: proteins, carbohydrates, sugar-free beverages, snacks, and condiments. I've also selected the 5 best choices for each category. These 25 foods are the building blocks for many of the recipes in this book. (See "5-Factor Recipes," page 110.) The beauty of the 5-Factor Must-Have Foods is that you can use your imagination and creativity, combining them to make your own quick and healthy meals that match the 5-Factor Diet formula.

THE 25 ESSENTIAL 5-FACTOR FOODS

Over the years I've figured out what works and what doesn't when it comes to diet. While there are no shortcuts in the pursuit of better nutrition and health, it is possible to keep your palate satisfied and your body in shape—and these 25 foods will help you do just that.

PROTEINS

1. Egg whites. Egg whites are often called the perfect source of protein because your body uses 100 percent of the nutrients they contain. They're also free of saturated fats, excess carbohydrates, and cholesterol, which many high-protein foods are laden with. But the main reason they rank high among my 5-Factor Must-Have Foods is the count-less ways you can cook them.

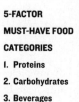

5-FACTOR
MUST-HAVE FOOD
CATEGORIES
I. Proteins
2. Carbohydrates
3. Beverages
4. Snacks
5. Condiments

Egg whites are easier than ever to use when cooking, especially since you no longer have to sep-arate them from the yolk yourself. Many grocery stores sell cartons of already-separated liquid egg whites. They're not only convenient but also pasteurized, so they last longer in the refrigerator and carry less risk of food poisoning.

My top picks: Eggology 100% Egg Whites and Egg Beaters Egg Whites

2. Poultry. I have only two rules when it comes to eating poultry: Choose white meat (which is leaner than dark meat) and remove the skin. Poultry is one of the few foods that you can easily strip fat from, so take full advantage of that perk. And remember that chicken isn't your only choice of poultry. Many people don't think of turkey except around the holidays, but it too is low in fat, high in protein, and loaded with ample amounts of zinc, iron, potassium phosphorus, and B vitamins.

To keep your taste buds interested, buy poultry in a variety of forms: Whole breasts are terrific, but so is ground poultry breast or sliced deli-style poultry (as long as it's all-natural and not heavily processed). Keep in mind that the packaged ground chicken and turkey you see in the grocery store often includes the skin so it can be as high in fat as ground beef. For that reason, it's best to have someone at the meat counter grind a skinless chicken or turkey breast for you.

Eva Mendes ACTRESS AND STAR OF THE MOVIE *HITCH*

"Harley has changed my life. Not only do I feel better than ever, but I now can have guilt-free pizza anytime, and that has made me a happy girl."

My top picks: I don't have a favorite brand, but I recommend that you become friendly with your local butcher. That way, you can specifically ask the butcher for the freshest and best cuts of poultry.

3. Seafood. Seafood should be a staple in every kitchen. Why? It's very low in fat and is packed with protein. Fish also contains healthy omega-3 fatty acids, which research has shown can improve the overall health of your heart, joints, and immune system. Better yet, seafood can have a mood-elevating effect on the brain by boosting levels of dopamine and serotonin, two neurotransmitters that naturally help prevent depression. The only downside of seafood is that some fish, specifically tuna, swordfish, and mackerel, may contain high levels of mercury. It's best to limit your intake of these to twice a week, except for light tuna, which you can have up to three times a week (see below).

My top picks: Salmon, cod, tuna, scallops, shrimp, lobster, squid, and crab. When buying canned tuna, pick the less-expensive versions (chunk light or flaked), which have less than half of the mercury of the more expensive white albacore variety. I love the convenience of StarKist Tuna Creations, which comes in a pouch instead of a can; it's easy to transport and easy to open, there's no water to drain, and it comes preflavored.

4. Dairy. Dairy has unfairly gotten a bad reputation because of its fat content, but it's an excellent source of protein and bone-strengthening calcium. Dairy also helps quell your appetite, according to researchers from the University of California at Davis. They found that study participants who ate meals containing dairy products had a 20 percent increase in an appetite-suppressing hormone called cholecystokinin.

Remember that dairy refers to more than just milk. It also comprises hard and soft cheeses (including cottage cheese and cream cheese), yogurt (plain with no sugar added), and sour cream. Always choose fat-free versions of these foods.

My top picks: Fat-free cheese slices, cottage cheese, and yogurt. When it comes to yogurt, stick to plain, non-fat, Greek-style yogurt from companies like Fage, Oikos, and Siggi's.

5. Game meats. While I was on a movie set a few years ago, I made a chili dinner for a few of the actors I was training. At the end of the meal, they all raved that it was the most delicious chili they'd ever eaten. It was only then that I revealed that the main ingredient was ground bison. They were stunned that its taste and texture were the same as those of regular beef—and thrilled that the fat content was about half that of beef.

Meats like ostrich, bison, elk, caribou, and venison may sound too exotic to eat, but *game* is actually a relative term. Go to the Far East and some of the more common meats are frog and turtle. Go to Eastern Europe and the Caribbean and it's not unusual to eat ox. So be daring and try game meats, which are often leaner than red meat, very high in protein, and high in iron. Adding them to your diet will make a big difference in your life because they let you enjoy the same tastes and textures as those of traditional beef and fat-laden steaks—without all the nutritional negatives.

Most health food and grocery stores stock game meats in their frozen section. Or look online for dealers that specialize in game meats.

There are two important things to remember when choosing game. One, make sure to read the nutritional label because certain cuts are leaner than others. Two, because game has less fat than regular beef, it's easy to overcook. Shave a few minutes off your usual cook time, or you could turn that bison steak into shoe leather.

My top pick: Intermountain Ostrich Cooperative ostrich burgers, Blackwing bison, Blackwing alligator, and Exotic Meats kangaroo loin fillet.

CARBS

1. Beans. Beans are mathematically a perfect food. Not only are they a low-glycemic carbohydrate with a small amount of healthy fats, but they're also high in protein and belly-filling fiber. In fact, one serving of beans (about ½ cup) provides close to 8 grams of fiber, which will leave you feeling more satiated—and less likely to overeat.

With so many varieties to choose from—black, red, kidney, pink, garbanzo, and many more—anyone can find a bean he or she likes. Beans are also perfect as a topping; sprinkle a handful on salads, chili, and soups to add extra fiber and protein to any meal.

My top picks: Most of the brands on the market are good, so pick whatever suits your taste buds. Studies have shown that canned beans have the same nutrient profile as fresh beans, so feel free to choose fresh, dried, frozen, or canned depending on what best fits your lifestyle.

2. Grains. Packed with fiber, grains are terrific because they fill you up and make a great companion to any protein. All forms of grain—including oatmeal, oats, lentils, barley, and brown rice—are good choices. One of my all-time favorites, however, is quinoa (pronounced "keen-wa"). This supergrain isn't a common staple—in fact, it can be difficult to find if your local grocery store doesn't have a large health food section—but it's loaded with about 50 percent more protein than most grains, and it's rich in calcium, iron, and the essential B vitamins.

My top picks: Kashi Golean cereal, Kashi 7 Whole Grain Pilaf, Quaker Weight Control instant oatmeal, Amy's organic lentil soup, and Eden Organic quinoa.

> **CARBS**
> 1. Beans
> 2. Grains
> 3. Breads
> 4. Vegetables
> 5. Fruit

3. Breads. I know what you're thinking: Bread is heavily processed, low in nutrients, and loaded with bad carbohydrates, so why is this a 5-Factor Must-Have Food? The problem with bread isn't bread itself but the ingredients that it's made from. I recommend that you avoid flour if possible. Luckily, there are several bread products such as tortillas, crackers, and flat bread that are made without flour. These products are made from sprouted grains that are not refined as much as flour. They're easy to spot because most brands will have the term *no-flour* or *flourless* right in the name of the product. These items may be located in the health food sec-

---

5-FACTOR DIET'S 5 FAVORITE VEGGIES

I. **Broccoli:** Just ½ cup of this superfood provides 66 percent of the Recommended Daily Allowance (RDA) of vitamin C and 10 percent of the RDA for vitamin A. It's also rich in potassium and fiber, which helps you feel fuller longer.

2. **Butternut squash:** This tasty veggie is more healthy than most people realize, with more than 80 percent of your RDA for vitamin A, 20 percent of the RDA for vitamin C, and almost 3 grams of fiber per ½-cup serving.

3. **Cauliflower:** Filled with vitamin A and belly-filling fiber, just ½ cup of cauliflower provides more than 33 percent of the RDA for vitamin C.

4. **Spinach:** It has everything: fiber, vitamins C and E, calcium, and folic acid, which is a vitamin that helps your body create healthy new cells.

5. **Sweet potato:** Loaded with vitamin C, ½ of a sweet potato yields close to 85 percent of the RDA for vitamin A.

---

tion of your supermarket. If your local stores don't carry no-flour breads, a second-best option is to choose breads made with whole grains.

My top picks: Fitness Bread by Mestemacher, Food for Life Ezekiel 4:19 Organic Sprouted Flourless Whole Grain Tortillas, Food for Life Ezekiel 4:19 Sprouted Whole Grain Flourless Cinnamon Raisin Bread

4. Vegetables. Low-calorie, low-glycemic, high in nutrients, and often packed with fiber, vegetables contain disease-fighting antioxidants (vitamins A and C) and potassium, which helps keep your muscles healthy. In short, you simply can't lead a healthy lifestyle if vegetables aren't a regular part of it. You can buy them fresh or frozen and eat them steamed, stir-fried, pureed, or grilled. Just remember that a healthy veggie quickly becomes unhealthy if it's batter-dipped or slathered with high-fat cheese sauce.

Which ones should you eat? Steer clear of avocados, olives, potatoes, and beets, which contain too much fat, carbohydrates, or sugars. All other vegetables are fair game. I prefer to buy mine frozen so I can stock up on all my favorites—and they will keep for months, unlike fresh veggies.

My top picks: Frozen mixed vegetables from Cascadian Farm or Westpac

5. Fruit. USDA research suggests that people who eat more fruit tend to have a lower body mass index (BMI) and lower total body weight than those who eat less fruit. Fruits are fat free and packed with fiber, vitamins, minerals, and antioxidants. Plus they let you enjoy sweet flavors without the empty calories of most sugary foods.

Not all fruits are equal. Some types—such as bananas—are higher on the glycemic index, which means they cause blood sugar levels to surge, thus triggering your body to store body fat. And you don't want that! Don't worry. Here's an easy way to remember which fruits rank low on the glycemic index and are therefore your best choices: The next time you pick up a piece of fruit, ask yourself these three questions. If you answer yes to at least one of them, it's a smart fruit choice:

Does it have edible skin?
(Think of apples, pears, plums, and peaches.)
Does it have edible seeds?
(Think of pomegranates, blackberries, strawberries, and raspberries.)
Is it a citrus fruit?
(Citrus fruits include grapefruit, oranges, and tangerines.)

The only exception to this rule is grapes, which do have an edible skin but are not a good fruit choice due to their high dextrose levels.

My top picks: Fresh fruit is best, but it's smart to keep a backup fruit handy in your freezer. Two of my favorites are Wyman's Quick-Frozen Mixed Fruit and Dole Mixed Berries.

BEVERAGES
1. Water. There's no better beverage than plain, unsweetened water. However, plain, flat water can get boring. To keep things interesting, I tell my clients to buy water in as many different forms as possible. Try sodium-free seltzer and, if you want to spice it up a bit and you're out for a night at a restaurant, sparkling water. Between all the bubbles and the fizz, sparkling water really helps cleanse the palate and adds a different texture.

My top picks: Bottled water (e.g. Dasani, Evian) and sparkling water (Pellegrino, Perrier)

2. Coffee. Coffee may sound like an odd choice for my 5-Factor Must-Have Foods, but there's a very important reason I include it. When I was a scientist for the Defense and Civil Institute of Environmental Medicine in Canada, I ran and published scientific studies on the effects of caffeine on exercise. Research has shown that drinking a caffeinated beverage 30 to 90 minutes before exercise can boost your endurance and increase the rate at which your body burns fat. Just keep an eye on how much coffee you drink—I would limit it to no more than three cups a day.

My top pick: Although I don't have a favorite brand, I prefer espresso beverages, such as cappucino and macchiatto. They typically have less than half the caffeine content of regular drip coffee and significantly more taste. The addition of nonfat milk to these beverages adds protein and calcium to your diet. My daily wake-up is usually nonfat espresso macchiatto.

If you do choose to drink regular coffee, keep a close watch on what you put in your cup. Ordinary plain coffee has no calories or sugar, but if you want to sweeten it up, I suggest using fat-free dairy products and Splenda.

3. Tea. Caffeinated tea is another must-have beverage because it offers the same endurance and metabolic benefits as coffee. But tea also comes with its own unique set of health advantages, so stock it in your kitchen, your desk drawer, and your purse or pocket so you always have a cup when you need it.

"I had a life-threatening illness and realized that to get through it, I needed to live a much healthier life. Because of its simplicity, 5-Factor allowed me to start while I was in treatment. The 5-Factor plan taught me how doing too much cardio and not eating enough of the right kinds of food combinations make your body hold on to the weight. All of the 5-Factor healthy eating habits helped me beat the illness, and I'm much healthier now."

Trina Jones AGE: **25** WEIGHT LOST SO FAR: **21 lbs.**

Certain teas—especially those that are rich in antioxidants such as polyphenols—have been shown to boost the immune system, ward off colds, soothe aches and pains, and even reduce the risk of developing cancer. One Rutgers University study found that TF-2, a component of black tea, kills colorectal cancer cells without affecting normal healthy cells in the body. The antioxidant polyphenols in some teas can even prevent heart disease. In 2003, USDA researchers found that subjects who drank five cups (there's that magic number again!) of black tea a day for three weeks lowered their LDL (bad) cholesterol by 11 percent.

BEVERAGES
1. Water
2. Coffee
3. Tea
4. Sugar-free soda
5. Sugar-free juices

As with coffee, drink no more than three cups of caffeinated tea daily. If you drink both coffee and tea, limit your daily consumption of both beverages to three cups total. Once you reach that limit, switch from caffeinated to decaffeinated teas and coffees.

My top picks: Black tea is terrific, but green tea also gets a lot of praise, for good reason. The polyphenols in this centuries-old beverage have been shown to fight certain cancers, ease pain, and burn calories. That's not bad for a few leaves and some water!

Any herbal tea will work fine too. Herbal teas are generally a combination of different herbs—not tea leaves—so they may not offer the same exact health benefits of tea. However, most are still calorie-free, contain different ratios of antioxidants, and offer health benefits that include everything from easing your stomach to relieving depression. Ice tea is a great option on a hot day. Try unsweetened Nestea, as it comes in many different flavors.

4. Sugar-free sodas. Most people enjoy an ice-cold soda, and that's entirely fine. Not all soda is bad for you. The problem with most sodas is that they are loaded with sugar—some have as much as 42 grams per serving—which can add 100 to 200 unwanted calories to your diet with every can or bottle. Instead, I recommend a no-calorie, Splenda-sweetened soda. That way, you'll stay hydrated and enjoy some flavor with your meal—without throwing on any extra calories. As part of the 5-Factor Diet, though, I would prefer that you limit yourself to one soda a day.

My top picks: Diet 7-Up, Diet Rite, and diet Hansen's Soda, which contains zero caffeine, no sugar, no preservatives, and no artificial flavors or coloring

5. Flavored waters. Like most sodas, many juice drinks contain excess sugar despite the fact that their product names sound healthy. That's why I recommend steering clear of any juices that have added sugar. All that sugar means excess calories that your body doesn't need.

My top picks: Fuze Slenderize tops my list, as it is sweetened with Splenda, is vitamin enhanced, and comes in a bunch of great flavors.

CONDIMENTS

1. Fat-free mayonnaise. Many healthy foods—such as tuna and certain vegetables—can be difficult to swallow because of their blandness. That's why fat-free mayo ranks high on the 5-Factor Must-Have Foods list. It's a "consistency" condiment, adding texture and taste to tuna dishes, chicken salad, salmon salad, and countless other meals.

If you stay away from fat-free mayonnaise because you don't like the taste, then you obviously haven't tried it in a while. Most of the fat-free brands available today actually taste good but without all the cholesterol and high amounts of saturated fat contained in regular mayo.

My top picks: Hellmann's Reduced Fat Mayonnaise and Kraft Fat-Free Mayo

2. Salsa. Just because you're used to eating salsa with bad-for-you foods like nachos doesn't mean this condiment should be banned from your eating routine. A healthy mix of tomatoes, onions, and other vegetables, salsa is all-natural, incredibly low in calories (as low as 4 calories per tablespoon), and a hands-down perfect substitute for high-fat dips and spreads. Salsa also contains lycopene, an antioxidant that may help prevent cancer, and it has absolutely no fat and only trace amounts of sodium.

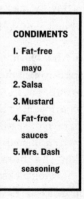

CONDIMENTS
1. Fat-free mayo
2. Salsa
3. Mustard
4. Fat-free sauces
5. Mrs. Dash seasoning

What I like most about salsa is that it has a zing that gives a kick to chili, soups, salads, or any other meal. Most salsas on the grocery store shelves are low calorie and low-fat. But shop wisely. You should still read the labels because a few of them have added sugar and higher calorie counts than you would expect. Avoid these at all costs!

My top picks: Pace salsas and Newman's Own salsas

3. Mustard. Mustard has three qualities that make it an ideal food: It adds consistency when mixed with other foods, it has a definite taste, and it's fat-free. (Stay away from mustards like honey mustard and Dijonnaise, which have more sugar and excess fat.) Whether you like it hot, spicy, regular, or yellow, mustard adds a sour or sweet spike, giving blander foods a bit of a kick.

My top pick: Gulden's Spicy Brown Mustard

4. Fat-free sauces. There are plenty of tasty sauces to choose from, but here are three that I highly recommend: soy, Worcestershire, and Tabasco. These are head and shoulders above the rest because they are practically calorie free—with no fat and no sugar—yet each packs a huge punch when it comes to adding tang, color, and flavor to foods. I find Worcestershire is an amazing sauce to perk up the flavor of soup as well as animal protein such as chicken or fish.

I'm not too concerned about whether you use a regular or low-sodium soy or Worcestershire sauce because most of the 5-Factor Must-Have Foods are low in sodium. Choose whichever one you think flavors your foods better.

If Tabasco is too intense for you, consider this: Research has shown that hot foods can mildly increase your metabolism. At the very least, a splash of Tabasco will encourage you to drink more water and fill up your belly even faster.

My top picks: 365 Organic Everyday Value Soy Ginger Sauce from Whole Foods Market and Lea & Perrins Worcestershire Sauce

5. Mrs. Dash. Why do I prefer this tried-and-true, sodium-free, sugar-free spice over all the other seasonings on the market? I'm not opposed to other brands, but I love that Mrs. Dash Seasoning Blend works with almost any food, making it the most versatile product I have in my kitchen. From fish and chicken to vegetables and soups, it's a great combination of herbs that turns even an amateur cook into a great chef. If you're not sure how to season something, just throw some Mrs. Dash on it and I guarantee it will taste terrific.

My top picks: The Mrs. Dash Original Blend is tasty, and it also comes in delicious flavors like Tomato Basil Garlic, Onion & Herb, Southwest Chipotle, and Extra Spicy. Include a few in your spice rack and you'll be ready to flavor up any meal.

SNACKS

1. Jerky. This superlean snack never needs to be refrigerated, so you can eat and transport it anywhere. Jerky is usually made with high-quality animal protein and very little fat or carbohydrates. With all the fat stripped out, you're left with pure, muscle-building protein—and no worries about the calories.

Because jerky is a cured meat, it can be high in sodium. I'm not too concerned about the sodium levels, given that most of the foods in the 5-Factor Diet are naturally low in sodium. (If you're concerned about your sodium intake, drink plenty of water each time you eat jerky.) However, you should watch out for sugar. Some brands use it to make their jerky sweet; you'll find it in barbecue-flavored jerky, for example. Stick with the regular-flavor varieties or others without excess sugar.

My top picks: Ostrim Ostrich Meat Sticks, Pemmican Turkey Jerky, and Pioneer Turkey Jerky

2. Oatmeal. A bowl of oats can help you maintain an even level of energy throughout the day, according to research from Penn State University. That's because oats are loaded with extra soluble fiber, which slows down the release of sugar into the bloodstream.

I prefer to buy boxes of individual-serving oatmeal packets so I can take and make it anywhere with just a little hot water. Read the labels if you're shopping for flavored oatmeal; it often has added sugar, which defeats the purpose of eating it. Look for flavored versions that are either sugar free or low in sugar.

My top picks: Quick Quaker Oats and Quaker Weight Control oatmeal, which has fiber and protein added, comes in flavors like apple-cinnamon and banana and is very low in sugar.

> **SNACKS**
> 1. Jerky
> 2. Oatmeal
> 3. Ready to
>   Drinks (RTD)
> 4. Veggie
>   meats
> 5. Non-flour
>   crackers

3. RTDs (Ready to Drinks). RTDs are meal replacement drinks that come in convenient cans and drink boxes or in a mixable powder form. Essentially RTDs are complete meals in liquid form, fortified with vitamins, minerals, and enough calories to help sustain you. They can be as filling as an average meal, thanks to a great mix of protein, carbohydrates, and fat. The only thing missing typically is fiber, which is why I tell people to consume a fruit or a fiber cracker when having an RTD.

A very important point to remember is that RTDs are not a "liquid diet." In "Fad Diets Don't Work," page 12, I told you that liquid diets—in which you typically substitute shakes for meals—fail mostly because the drinks are basically water with just enough sugar to keep you barely functioning. RTDs are completely different. I think they're perfect, especially as an on-the-go snack, but certainly not as a replacement for several meals in a row.

My top picks: Lean Body Ready-to-Drink Shakes or RTDs from Met-Rx and Myoplex

4. Veggie Meats. Veggie dogs, veggie burgers, veggie bologna—today's grocery stores sell a wide assortment of faux meat products. They're smart substitutes for the real things because they contain very little fat, are typically as high in protein as real meat, and are extremely low in carbohydrates. They are also ideal to keep on hand in your fridge because they stay fresh as long as a month, which is a lot longer than fresh chicken, beef, or fish. If you doubt that they'll satisfy your taste buds, trust me when I say that food manufacturers have finally perfected the art of turning vegetables into a food that has all the flavor of real meat.

It's worth remembering that vegetarian meat isn't always healthier than regular meat. Certain brands of veggie burgers and veggie dogs are much higher in fat than I prefer. I suggest that you stick to products that are high in protein and get less than 20 percent of their calories from fat.

My top pick: Yves Veggie Cuisine products

5. No-flour Crackers and Brown Rice Cakes. No-flour crackers, made with whole grains instead of flour have roughly 5 grams of healthy fiber and less than 2 grams of fat per serving. Brown rice cakes are fat-free. These low-fat snacks are what I call the perfect "transport mechanism" for protein. Stack some turkey or smoked salmon on top and you'll get a high-protein, low-glycemic snack with a great crunch.

You'll find no-flour crackers and brown rice cakes in the health food section of your supermarket or right next to the less-healthy, flour-packed crackers and regular rice cakes.

When buying non-flour crackers, always check the list of ingredients on the package. You shouldn't find the word *flour* in any form—no flour, rice flour, wheat flour, rye flour, etc. Also look for the word *oil*. If you can find a brand with neither flour nor oil, you have a winner.

My top picks: Bran-a-crisp crackers, Quaker Rice Cakes (regular size)

5-FACTOR MUST-HAVE FOODS SHOPPING CHECKLIST

These are my celebrity clients' go-to foods. Now they're all yours. To be sure that you always have these 25 essential foods in your kitchen, copy this page and post it on your fridge. Shop so that you have at least one week's worth of each item in your home at all times.

PROTEINS
- ☐ Egg Whites
- ☐ Poultry
- ☐ Seafood
- ☐ Dairy
- ☐ Game

CONDIMENTS
- ☐ Fat-Free Mayo
- ☐ Salsa
- ☐ Mustard
- ☐ Fat-Free Sauces
- ☐ Mrs. Dash

CARBS
- ☐ Beans
- ☐ Grains
- ☐ Breads
- ☐ Vegetables
- ☐ Fruit

SNACKS
- ☐ Jerky
- ☐ Oatmeal Packets
- ☐ Ready To Drinks (RTDs)
- ☐ Veggie Meats
- ☐ No-flour Crackers

SUGAR-FREE BEVERAGES
- ☐ Water
- ☐ Coffee
- ☐ Tea
- ☐ Sugar-Free Juice
- ☐ Sugar-Free Soda

CHAPTER 8

Shopping for 5-Factor Foods

One of the greatest challenges of following any diet program is figuring out exactly how to incorporate it into your personal day-to-day routine. In this chapter, I'm going to show you how seamless the transition to a healthy lifestyle can be. An important part of this is rethinking your relationship with your grocery store. Being a smarter, savvier, healthier shopper just takes a little understanding about all the foods vying for your attention.

SMART WAYS TO NAVIGATE A GROCERY STORE
Sticking to the 5-Factor Diet requires you to make healthy choices, but that's not always easy to do when visiting the supermarket. How you shop and where you shop play a big role in whether you'll cheat on your diet. Use my 5-Factor shopping rules to ensure that every trip to the market is a healthy one.

1. SHOP EARLY

Even if you're not a morning person, make an effort to do your grocery shopping early in the day. Your body will thank you for it. Getting to the market early offers more than just avoiding the late-afternoon crowd—you'll also have your pick of the freshest foods available because most markets set out their produce and fresh meats in the morning. You can pick the best cuts of meat and choicest fruits and vegetables, thereby increasing your odds of choosing foods that are still packed with nutrients. Shop later in the day and you'll be stuck with older foods that have been picked through and, most likely, have lost nutrients.

> **5-FACTOR GROCERY STORE RULES**
> I. Shop early.
> 2. Go with a full stomach.
> 3. Stick to the outside aisles.
> 4. Always have a plan.
> 5. Shop at the same store.

2. GO WITH A FULL STOMACH

Shopping for food when you're hungry is a recipe for disaster because your body desperately craves anything to fill its void, preferably something high in sugar and fat. That's why you should shop right after your first meal (breakfast) or your second meal (midmorning snack). That way, you'll feel satiated and be less tempted to pick up foods that aren't good for you.

3. STICK TO THE OUTSIDE AISLES

Most grocery stores share similar layouts, keeping their most healthy and nutritious foods around the perimeter. Do a lap around the store—going in one big rectangle—and you'll likely find almost all the foods on the 5-Factor Diet, including your produce, dairy, and meats. Avoid the inside aisles as much as possible; this is where you'll find most of the foods that are higher in fat and lower in nutrients. The only exception to this rule is the frozen food aisle, which is usually not on the perimeter. This is one of my favorite aisles when shopping for the 5-Factor Diet. (See "The Frozen Food Aisle is A Dieter's Best Friend," page 66.)

4. ALWAYS HAVE A PLAN

Never go to the supermarket without a well-thought-out list. Without a clear plan, you're more likely to buy bad foods on impulse. You may also forget to buy enough 5-Factor Foods. Remember, you need to eat foods from all five 5-Factor categories at each meal in order to achieve the best results, so missing even one of the five will hold back your progress.

I know you're busy, so simply copy the "5-Factor Must-Have Foods Shopping Checklist" on page 63 and you'll guarantee that you always have the right 5-Factor Diet foods in your kitchen.

5. SHOP AT THE SAME STORE
Once you find a store that carries all of the 5-Factor Diet foods, avoid frustration and shop only at that one store whenever possible. Being familiar with the layout of a store makes it much easier to get what you need quickly and avoid the aisles with bad foods. If you're regularly popping into unfamiliar supermarkets, you'll increase your risk of getting lost and walking past unhealthy goodies that may tempt you.

THE FROZEN FOOD AISLE IS A DIETER'S BEST FRIEND
Most dieters shy away from the frozen food aisle—and why wouldn't they? It's home to some of the most tempting, fattening foods around, from ice cream and frozen pizzas to those man-size TV dinners whose packaging has more nutrients than the actual food inside. If dieters do venture into this aisle, they probably zip past all the frozen desserts en route to the packaged—and pricey—diet meals put out by Healthy Choice and Weight Watchers. If this sounds like you, then you're missing out on all the great things the frozen food aisle has to offer—especially when it comes to implementing the 5-Factor Diet.

Every food has some sort of nutritional value, but its protein, vitamins, and minerals have a shelf life. From the moment a food is picked, caught, or killed, a nutritional clock starts ticking. Everything that happens to the food from that point forward ages it, affecting how much nutritional value you'll get from it when it finally finds its way to your mouth. As more people handle the food, the risk of it being tainted by things like bacteria or viruses increases. Every person that touches the food causes more bruising, which can make it spoil faster. The longer a food sits in a box or on a truck, the more it deteriorates. Even exposure to sunlight can degrade some of the important nutrients.

That's why the frozen food aisle is the 5-Factor dieter's greatest ally. Here are my top five reasons why you should no longer fear the frozen food aisle.

1. YOU GET MORE NUTRIENTS

When you buy frozen foods such as fruits and vegetables, they are flash-frozen almost immediately after they're harvested, so fewer people handle them. They're usually sealed in packages that are impervious to light. Time essentially stops, leaving all of the foods' nutrients sealed inside.

This means that when you buy a frozen strawberry at the grocery store, it's as nutritionally fresh as the day it was picked. After a good thaw, it is young and delicious again. On the other hand, a fresh strawberry in the produce aisle has an unknown history. It may have been picked out of state, then sifted, sorted, crated, warehoused, packaged, and trucked to a distribution center before being delivered to your local grocer and put out for display. It may have sat for as long as 10 days being touched by strangers and exposed to light. By the time you eat it, that strawberry is old. In fact, the FDA and the USDA have compared many fresh fruits and vegetables against frozen versions and found the two have relatively equivalent nutrient

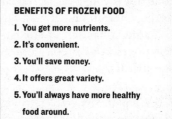

BENEFITS OF FROZEN FOOD

1. You get more nutrients.
2. It's convenient.
3. You'll save money.
4. It offers great variety.
5. You'll always have more healthy food around.

profiles. In fact, in some cases, certain nutrient levels are higher in the frozen foods.

2. IT'S CONVENIENT

I love raw vegetables, but sometimes a bag of frozen mixed veggies or stir-fry veggies is more convenient. Fresh vegetables require a lot of cleaning and chopping. With frozen veggies, all that hard work has been done for you. Just grab a bag of mixed vegetables and they're ready to be added to a stir-fry or made into a side dish. Frozen meats and fish are even more of a time-saver. With no cleaning involved, just thaw and you're ready to cook—mess free!

3. YOU'LL SAVE MONEY

A lot of my clients think frozen foods are more expensive, but ask yourself this: How many times have you thrown away fresh chicken, fish, fruits, or vegetables because they sat around in your fridge too long? We've all done it. With frozen foods, you rarely have to throw anything away because it has spoiled; most foods stay fresh for months in the freezer.

4. IT OFFERS GREAT VARIETY

I'm big on berries, but they aren't in season as often as I'd like. Luckily, I can always find them in the frozen food aisle, along with any other out-of-season fruits I may be craving.

I recommend you keep a big bag of stir-fry vegetables in the freezer. Why? Because a lot of dieters stick with eating the same veggies over and over again. Don't get me wrong; eating vegetables is good, but different vegetables often have different amounts of vitamins and minerals. If you're eating the same one or two vegetables, you may be getting a lot of, say, vitamin A while missing out on iron or vitamin C. Eating a handful of stir-fry veggies (I like to steam them) gives you an assortment every time, so you're guaranteed a balanced mix of nutrients.

5. YOU'LL ALWAYS HAVE HEALTHY FOOD AROUND

Having lots of healthy food around is terrific, but it's not always practical to buy a 10-pound tray of fresh chicken breasts from the meat department! But you can find these foods in the frozen aisle, along with fruits and vegetables that come in 5- to 10-pound bags. Buying in bulk may seem like a space eater in your freezer, but it works to your advantage. It guarantees that you'll always have healthy foods to eat (and less space

---

TIPS FOR BUYING FROZEN FOODS

1. Buy vegetables raw—and never with cheese sauce or butter packets!

2. Before buying fruit, read the label. The only ingredient should be the fruit itself, not syrup.

3. When you pick up meat, gently squeeze the package. If you hear or feel a crunch, it's probably freezer-burned.

4. Always reach into the back of the freezer, where food is kept colder.

5. Read the cooking instructions. Some frozen foods are precooked, which means you could be getting more sugars and bad fats than if they were raw.

to stock unhealthy options). By keeping the freezer well stocked, you'll never run out and be left reaching for something off the 5-Factor Diet when you're hungry.

PICKING THE BEST SWEETENERS

When you shop for healthy foods, you'll come across many low- or reduced-calorie foods. They may sound good, but it's important to know exactly what natural or artificial substitute you're eating in place of sugar. Some of these sweeteners may be great for adding calorie-free flavor to your food, but many come with health issues of which you should be aware.

THE SEVEN MOST COMMON SUGAR SUBSTITUTES

I have to break from my use of the number 5 for a moment because we need to examine seven common sweeteners used today: sucrose, turbinado, honey, aspartame, saccharin, sucralose (Splenda), and stevia. You should make your own personal decision about which sweeteners to use, based on the facts about these products, including what the manufacturers won't tell you. Here's the truth—and my recommendations—about sweeteners.

> "My biggest problem was finding a diet that accommodated my busy schedule. Between work, travel, and my family, I had no time to get in shape. Your diet was so simple to follow, with suitable food choices and simple substitutions. The rapid changes I experienced only increased my motivation to succeed. Thank you!"
>
> **David Widman, M.D.** AGE: 41 WEIGHT LOST: 15 lbs. in 4 weeks

Sucrose (or sugar). Sucrose is the most common food sweetener in the world. Extracted from sugar cane or sugar beets, it's purified and crystallized, then stripped of all vitamins, minerals, fiber, amino acids, and trace elements. It may be nutritionally worthless, but because of its taste and the quick hit of energy it provides, sugar is a hard habit to kick.

Unfortunately, the fleeting burst of energy usually disappears as quickly as it came, leaving you feeling more sluggish than you did before eating. This effect is called "reactive hypoglycemia." Think of it this way: Eating sugar is like accelerating your car by flooring the gas, then taking your foot off the pedal and letting the car go back to its normal speed. At a certain point, your car will slow down to the speed at which it was running before you hit the gas, then slow down even further (and eventually stop altogether). When you eat sugar, your energy levels ultimately dip below your baseline, which is why you end up craving even more sugar later.

It's a vicious cycle, and it's the reason why we obsess about sweet foods. But our consumption comes at a price. Just like highly glycemic carbohydrates, sugar causes an insulin surge that makes your body store calories as fat—even if you're eating fat-free sweets. Research has shown that sugar has the same effect as other carbohydrates on blood sugar levels. Calorie for calorie, sugar raises blood glucose about the same amount as starches such as white bread and white potatoes.

Turbinado. You may not recognize its real name, but you've seen it in the light brown packets. It's that dark brown, coarse, "raw" sugar that's supposed to be better for you because it's all-natural and chemical free. (White table sugar, by comparison, is processed with things like phosphoric acid, sulphur dioxide, and bleaching agents, to name just a few!) Turbinado is usually made by squeezing the juice out of crushed sugar cane, then spinning what's left after evaporation through a huge centrifuge. Because it's not chemically treated, it's supposed to be richer in vitamins and minerals.

Wrong! The big mistake most people make is assuming that turbinado is healthier than table sugar because it's unbleached. This assumption causes some people to use even more of it than they would regular sugar. People make a similar mistake when comparing white bread with breads that are dyed brown to seem more natural. But just because something is darker doesn't always mean it's better for you! White sugar and dark sugar may have different characteristics and tastes, but your body reacts to both in the same way, with a fat-storing insulin spike.

Honey. I don't recommend honey. Honey producers make a lot of healthy promises, claiming honey can protect you against cancer and heart disease because it contains antioxidants and certain enzymes. The problem is, honey—no matter how unrefined and all-natural its producers may say it is—is still nothing more than pure sugar. To be exact, it's an invert sugar— created by an enzyme in bee nectar—that's an extremely dense, gelatinous form of easily absorbed sugar. At best, honey has only trace amounts of antioxidants, vitamins, and minerals. That's true whether you're talking about buckwheat honey, sunflower honey, or regular clover honey.

Honey should never take the place of fruits and veggies, which are far richer in antioxidants and have much less sugar. You get far more antioxidants and nutrients from a single piece of fruit than you ever could from pouring on honey and adding excess sugar to your diet. It's the wrong approach.

Aspartame. You may know it by other names (such as NutraSweet or Equal), but aspartame is a low-calorie sweetener that is about 200 times sweeter than sugar. However, it's not the best sweetener for use in hot drinks or cooking because it tends to lose its sweetness in high temperatures. That's why coffee or tea drinkers who use aspartame may find themselves pouring in extra packets when reaching for their morning pick-me-up.

There is a great deal of controversy over this sweetener, especially because it's made from methyl alcohol, which on its own is potentially toxic. Despite that, aspartame has been proven safe for human consumption. However, people with a rare hereditary metabolic condition called phenylketonuria (PKU) need to watch their intake of aspartame because it contains the enzyme phenylalanine, which they must avoid. That's why some product labels print "This product contains phenylalanine" on them. If you're pregnant, avoid aspartame because it's impossible to know if your baby has PKU.

Personally, I don't like the taste of aspartame but if you want to use it, I would prefer that you have it in small amounts only.

WHAT IS "PERCENT DAILY VALUE"?

Understanding Percent Daily Values—which is often shortened to "% Daily Value" or "%DV"—is key to deciphering any food label. These percentages tell you how a single serving of the food fits into a typical 2,000-calorie-a-day meal plan. (If you consume more or less than 2,000 calories, you need to adjust the Percent Daily Value accordingly.) At a glance, you can tell whether a food is high or low in a specific nutrient. For example, the label might tell you that a food provides 13% of your recommended daily value of carbohydrates or 35% of your fats. It's also a snap to compare the nutrients in products against each other—just be sure the serving sizes match first.

Sugars, protein, and trans fats don't have a Percent Daily Value, so you won't see a percentage listed for them. The FDA hasn't determined yet how much protein the average person should consume daily. As for sugar and trans fats, the FDA doesn't want you eating either, so it naturally doesn't recommend any set amount.

Saccharin. Sweet'N Low and Sugar Twin are two brands of saccharin you're most likely familiar with. Saccharin is so popular because it can sweeten both hot and cold foods and is low calorie. Some people have had concerns about the sweetener because older studies found that rats who ingested large amounts of the sweetener were at risk for cancer. New research has found saccharin is safe in the small amounts most people use. But I'll be honest with you—I'm not a big saccharin fan. In fact, following a 1977 study in which rats got bladder cancer after being fed saccharin, Canada, where I am originally from, banned it from being sold. It still is not sold there, which should say something in itself. If you choose to use saccharin in lieu of sugar, I recommend the smallest amounts possible, just to be safe.

Stevia. Stevia is a natural dietary supplement extracted from the *Stevia rebaudiana* plant, and it has been used for decades around the world, especially in Japan. It's about 300 times sweeter than sugar and is calorie-free. Go to any health food store and you'll see it touted as the most popular natural alternative to sugar. However, the FDA hasn't approved it for use as a sweetener. Why not? A few studies have shown that stevia may cause cancer and reproductive health problems, which is why Canada and some other countries won't allow it to be used as a sweetener. The FDA does state that when used sparingly, stevia is perfectly safe—although the agency believes it could create health issues if approved as an artificial sweetener. Stevia is definitely an acquired taste; it can change the flavor of foods and beverages.

Sucralose (Splenda). Sucralose is 600 times sweeter than sugar and the newest low-calorie sweetener on the market—and is my sweetener of choice. It's basically regular table sugar that's been chlorinated, a process that tweaks it just enough so that it doesn't make your blood sugar rise. It also retains its sweetness in hot and cold foods.

To this point, there haven't been any negative findings in research on sucralose usage. In Canada, we've been using it for about 15 years.

DECIPHERING FOOD LABELS

Before I start working with clients, I give them reading material about nutrition. We talk everything through and I teach them how to cook, whether they want to or not. If they want to taste my food, they have to watch me cook it. Why? Because I want to empower them. Once they understand how their bodies work with the foods they eat, following the 5-Factor Diet is even easier. They gain a sense of confidence in the program, even when I'm not there. They can follow my advice without having to question why it works.

WHAT TO EXPECT ON A FOOD LABEL

SERVING SIZE
SERVINGS PER CONTAINER
CALORIES
 Calories from fat
TOTAL FAT
 Saturated fat
 Trans fat
 Polyunsaturated fat
 Monounsaturated fat
CHOLESTEROL
SODIUM
TOTAL CARBOHYDRATES
 Dietary fiber
 Sugars
 Other carbohydrates
PROTEIN
VITAMINS AND MINERALS
 Vitamin A
 Vitamin C
 Calcium
 Iron
 Vitamin D
 Thiamin
 Riboflavin
 Niacin
 Vitamin B_6
 Phosphorus
 Magnesium
 Zinc
LESS THAN SERIES
LIST OF INGREDIENTS

A lot of diet books tell you what to eat and maybe a little bit about why you should eat that way. But they don't empower you to make good choices for yourself. Being able to decipher what's in every single food gives you power. You can finally look through your fridge and cupboards and understand—maybe for the first time in your life—what will work and what won't work for your diet.

WHAT YOU NEED TO KNOW

In this book you're already learning the science of nutrition. How you apply that knowledge starts with understanding the foods you eat. That's why knowing how to read a nutritional label is one of the most important lessons I can teach you. Here's the information you'll find on the label— and what those numbers mean to you.

Serving size. This number tells you what quantity of the food was used to determine the nutrition facts. To make it easy for you to compare it to other, similar foods, the measurements are usually standard: The label will first list the serving size in lay terms (such as ½ cup or 6 pieces), then give you the metric amount (122 grams, for example).

5-Factor Fact: Most people eat a lot more than the recommended serving size. Try portioning out one serving size to get a better sense of how many servings you're really eating when you have that food.

Servings per container. This number tells you the approximate number of servings the package contains.

5-Factor Fact: This information is amazingly helpful. Some foods have very small serving sizes so that the amount of calories per serving seems low. That is, until you do the math. Multiplying the "servings per container" by "calories per serving" will give you the caloric content of the entire package.

Calories and calories from fat. In addition to telling you how many calories you're getting per serving, the label also shows exactly how many of those calories are from fat.

5-Factor Fact: Seeing big numbers in the "calories from fat" section shouldn't always scare you. Good-for-you fats such as olive oil get *all* of their calories from fat.

Total fat. This number combines the fat grams from all four types of fats: saturated, trans, polyunsaturated, and monounsaturated.

    5-Factor Fact: The FDA suggests that you eat no more than 65 grams of fat per day.

Saturated fat. This is the number of saturated fat grams contained in each serving.

    5-Factor Fact: Your daily maximum of this unhealthy fat is 20 grams, according to the FDA. I suggest keeping your intake of this dangerous fat even lower.

Trans fat. This shows how many grams of trans fat are in each serving.

    5-Factor Fact: In January 2006, the FDA began requiring all food manufacturers to list trans fat on their labels. That's good news because

---

Alicia Keys GRAMMY-WINNING SINGER/SONGWRITER

"Harley's style of working out is 100 percent my style. It doesn't take a lot of time out of your day, it's motivating, and you feel good (especially when people take notice!). The focus is not on starving yourself but on healthful living, so you don't feel like you're missing out on the foods you love. Once you get started, you get addicted to looking, feeling, and living your best."

GOOD NEWS FOR ALLERGY SUFFERERS

Each year approximately 30,000 people in the United States require emergency room treatment and 150 die because of allergic reactions to food. Now, new food label laws may help prevent some of these problems. In January 1, 2006, the FDA began requiring that food labels clearly identify when ingredients contain protein derived from the eight major allergenic foods: milk, eggs, fish, crustacean shellfish, tree nuts, peanuts, wheat, and soybeans. If you're allergic to these foods, read the list of ingredients; you should find any troublesome ingredient listed along with the source of the food allergen.

before this it was tough to determine what foods contained this dangerous form of fat. Don't expect to find a Percent Daily Value listed for this bad-for-you fat, because your body doesn't need it. Keep your consumption of trans fat as close to zero as possible.

Polyunsaturated fat. This is the total number of polyunsaturated fat grams per serving.

5-Factor Fact: Unlike saturated fat, polyunsaturated fat doesn't raise cholesterol levels. Rather, it actually lowers the amount of bad cholesterol lipids, called low-density lipoproteins (LDLs).

Monounsaturated fat. This is the total number of monounsaturated fat grams in each serving.

5-Factor Fact: Olive oil is an excellent source of monounsaturated fat, plus it makes a great base for salad dressing.

Cholesterol. This is the total milligrams of cholesterol per serving.

5-Factor Fact: Although your body needs cholesterol to assist with hormone production and other bodily functions, your liver manufactures cholesterol on its own. That's why you should limit your daily intake to 300 milligrams.

Sodium. This is the total milligrams of sodium per serving.

5-Factor Fact: I'm not overly concerned about excess sodium in the diet because only a very small percentage of the population is sodium sensitive. Sodium is relatively benign and passes out of the body

> "For me, starting a new program was less about losing a bunch of weight and more about wanting to finally tone and shape my middle-age body. My butt and thighs were beginning to make a world of their own! I didn't understand which foods were beneficial and which ones should simply be avoided, but the nutrition explanations in 5-Factor taught me what I should aim for with each and every meal."
>
> **Mashell Smith** AGE: **44** WEIGHT LOST SO FAR: **7 lbs.**

fairly quickly. The FDA recommends keeping your daily intake below 2,400 milligrams. Of course, if you have high blood pressure or kidney issues, then you should monitor your sodium intake more closely.

Total carbohydrates. This number is the total grams of every type of carbohydrate—dietary fiber, sugars, and other sources—per serving.
   5-Factor Fact: The FDA suggests a daily total carb consumption of 300 grams or less. As you already know, I want you to eat only carbs with low to moderate glycemic levels. But food labels don't tell you what the carbohydrates' glycemic level is. To find out, go to the glycemic index database at www.glycemicindex.com.

Dietary fiber. This is how many grams of fiber—both soluble and insoluble—are in each serving. This amount is included in the total carbohydrates measurement, but dietary fiber affects blood sugar less than other types of carbs do. That's why the American Diabetes Association suggests that if a food has 5 grams or more of fiber per serving, you can subtract this number from the carbohydrate total.

5-Factor Fact: Fiber comes in two types—soluble and insoluble—but nutrition labels aren't required to list them separately. However, most manufacturers will tell you somewhere on the package how many grams of insoluble fiber their product contains.

Sugars. This is where you'll see how many grams of sugar are in each serving. You may also see "sugar alcohols" or "sugar replacers" listed. Sugar alcohols don't affect your blood sugar levels as much as sugar does, but they have a caloric value 10 percent greater than other carbs.

5-Factor Fact: If you see grams of sugar on the nutrition label but can't find the word *sugar* on the list of ingredients, that's because sugar sometimes goes by different names. Check the list for names like fructose (fruit sugar), glucose (dextrose), galactose (milk sugar), lactose (a combination of glucose and galactose), and maltose (malt sugar).

Other carbohydrates. This number—which isn't on all labels—is a catch-all category for any other types of carbohydrates that may be in each serving.

5-Factor Fact: These trace carbs—typically various organic acids and flavenoids—don't raise your blood sugar level very much, so don't be concerned about them. Sometimes sugar alcohols are thrown into this category as well; sugar alcohols may include malitol, sorbitol, xylitol, and glycerine.

Protein. This is how many grams of protein are in each serving.

5-Factor Fact: Sometimes dairy protein appears on an ingredient list in the form of albumen, whey, or casein.

Vitamin and mineral percentages. All food labels are required to list vitamin A, vitamin C, calcium, and iron content. Other nutrients—such as vitamin D, thiamin, riboflavin, niacin, vitamin B6, phosphorus, magnesium, and zinc—are shown only if they're added as a supplement.

You won't see how many grams or milligrams of each nutrient are in a serving. Instead you'll see what percentage of the recommended daily amount of that nutrient is contained in each serving.

Ingredients. Finally, a label lists all the food's ingredients, arranged in descending order based on the weight of each ingredient.

5-Factor Fact: Because of the ranking of ingredients by weight, the first few ingredients listed are typically the bulk of what's in the food. For a real eye-opener, compare the ingredients list of a processed food with its natural equivalent—for instance, processed, sugary fruit drink versus 100 percent fresh-squeezed juice. The differences will startle you.

Tracee Ross
ACTRESS AND STAR ON THE
TV SHOW *GIRLFRIENDS*

"Harley has taught me to love my body in a way I haven't since I was 18. I just want to run around naked with a tattoo on my ass that says, "Body by Harley." Harley has taught me how to keep myself toned, lean, and strong and still have that perfect amount of womanly jiggle so I look and feel good on and off screen. Since I met Harley, I am never more than two weeks from my ideal."

LEARN THE LINGO

If you see this word ...	Then the food contains ...
LEAN	Less than 10 grams of fat, 4 grams of saturated fat, and 95 milligrams of cholesterol.
EXTRA LEAN	Less than 5 grams of fat, 2 grams of saturated fat, and 95 milligrams of cholesterol.
REDUCED FAT	25% less fat than the regular version.
MORE	At least 10% more of a specific nutrient, compared to the regular version.
GOOD SOURCE OF	10–19% of the Daily Value of a particular nutrient.
HIGH IN	20% or more of the Daily Value recommended for that particular nutrient.
LIGHT OR LITE	At least one-third fewer calories than the regular version of that food, or no more than half of the fat. If you see the word in reference to sodium, it means the food has at least 50% less sodium than the regular version.

If you see this word ...	Then the food contains ...
LOW	Less of a particular nutrient per serving than the regular version of that food. How much less depends on the nutrient.
	If a food is "low calorie," it has less than 40 calories per serving.
	If a food is "low fat," it has less than 3 grams of total fat per serving.
	If a food is "low in saturated fat," it has less than I gram of saturated fat per serving.
	If a food is "low cholesterol," it has less than 20 milligrams of cholesterol per serving.
	If a food is "low sodium," it has less than 140 milligrams of sodium per serving.
	If a food is "very low sodium," it has less than 35 milligrams per serving.
FREE	Little or no trace of a particular nutrient per serving.
	If a food is "calorie-free," it has less than 5 calories per serving.
	If a food is "fat-free" it has less than 0.5 gram of total fat per serving.
	If a food is "free of saturated fat," it has less than 0.5 gram of saturated fat per serving.
	If a food is "cholesterol-free," it has less than 2 milligrams of cholesterol per serving.
	If a food is "sodium-free," it has less than 5 milligrams of sodium per serving.
	If a food is "sugar-free," it has less than 0.5 gram of sugars per serving.
% FAT-FREE	This designates the actual amount of a food that is not made up of fat. But don't be fooled. A product may be "90% fat-free," but the other 10% might be loaded in calories.
REDUCED	At least 25% less of a nutrient, compared to the regular product.

CHAPTER 9

New 5-Factor Hollywood Workout

You can't transform your body through diet alone.

Burning fat, shaping your muscles, feeling better, and being healthier—it all starts with a smart eating plan and an equally smart exercise program. Other diets "suggest" exercise without giving specifics, or they prescribe a regimen that's too complex or too time-consuming for anyone with a life. The 5-Factor program is not like any other diet you've ever tried.

My first book, *5-Factor Fitness*, focused more on exercise, while in this book I've been able to give you more nutritional information and exciting, delicious recipes to try. Still, exercise remains a major component of my program if you want the best results possible.

If you have my first book, you're in for a treat. The exercises and routines in this chapter are all new, yet equally effective, so you'll build even more lean muscle tissue and burn off even more body fat. I'll also show you how to extend the original five-week workout plan into a five-month fitness regime that will truly take your body to the next level. If you're brand-new to exercise and 5-Factor fitness, don't worry. My plan is the easiest, most effective exercise program you'll ever use.

5-FACTOR HOLLYWOOD WORKOUT SECRETS

The 5-Factor Hollywood Workout routine, just like my 5-Factor Diet, is simple: You'll do 5 workouts a week, each 25 minutes long and broken into the following five 5-minute phases:

Phase 1: 5 minutes of cardio warm-up
Phase 2: 5 minutes of upper-body strength training
Phase 3: 5 minutes of lower-body strength training
Phase 4: 5 minutes of core training
Phase 5: 5 minutes of fat-burning cardio work

That's it. If you can give me—or should I say, your body—125 minutes total of attention each week for a recommended five-week cycle, your results will amaze you.

With the 5-Factor Diet's 5-phase workout, I've had clients lose 5 or more pounds a month, without ever feeling like they're spending all their time working out. In fact, by tweaking the final cardio portion of the workout, you can burn off even more body fat, as I'll explain when I describe Phase 5 in detail.

I'm sure you're wondering how a workout that takes so little time can be so effective. You shouldn't be surprised that I have five very good reasons!

1. IT NEVER LETS YOUR MUSCLES REST

The 5-Factor Hollywood Workout uses an advanced technique called

5-FACTOR WORKOUT SECRETS
1. It never lets your muscles rest.
2. It's more intense.
3. It targets more muscle fibers.
4. It's perfectly balanced.
5. It makes you do more reps.

"supersetting," in which you do two exercises back-to-back without resting in between. This makes the workout shorter but keeps your heart rate elevated longer, so you burn more calories.

2. IT'S MORE INTENSE

Most workout routines have you perform exercises exactly the same way every time. For instance, you may be asked to do three sets of 12 repetitions per exercise, with 60 seconds of rest between sets. The 5-Factor Workout, on the other hand, constantly changes the type of exercise, the number of repetitions, the rest time between super-sets, and the resistance level of your workout. Because the workout is constantly changing, your body never gets bored so it keeps evolving, keeps burning fat, and never stops progressing.

3. IT TARGETS MORE MUSCLE FIBERS

Many workouts you see in magazines string together exotic exercises that isolate only specific, small muscle groups. The problem with that approach? To burn the most calories, you have to involve as many muscles as possible.

That's why the 5-Factor Workout targets large muscle groups, such as your chest, back, quadriceps, and hamstrings, twice a week. Smaller muscle groups, such as your biceps, triceps, and shoulders, get a workout once a week.

4. IT'S PERFECTLY BALANCED

The muscles on the front of your body (chest, biceps, quadriceps) work in tandem with the muscles on the back of your body (back, triceps, and hamstrings). Most routines don't account for that fact, and they end up working one side of the body more than the other. With the 5-Factor Hollywood Workout, you work opposing muscle groups equally, so your body gets a balanced workout.

5. IT MAKES YOU DO MORE REPS

Other routines call for 8 to 12 repetitions of each exercise—or maybe go as high as 15. The 5-Factor Hollywood Workout pushes your muscles beyond average levels of fatigue by sometimes requiring 15 to 25 reps. This technique uses more calories, so you end up burning off even more body fat.

THE 5 PHASES OF THE 5-FACTOR HOLLYWOOD WORKOUT

My workout breaks down into 5 phases, each of which lasts for 5 minutes. You'll always start with Phase 1, then move to Phase 2, then Phase 3, then Phase 4, and finish with Phase 5. From start to finish, the routine takes only 25 minutes. To give your body a chance to recover, you'll exercise five days a week and incorporate a rest day twice a week. (In this book, I've made Wednesday and Sunday rest days; feel free to choose whichever two days are best for your schedule.) To get the best results, follow my 5-week program, which builds up intensity gradually so that by week 5, your body is burning calories at its highest possible pace.

PHASE 1: 5-MINUTE CARDIO WARM-UP

Warm up with 5 minutes of light cardio exercise. You can walk, cycle, stair climb, or use a cardio machine set on a low level. It doesn't matter what you do because the goal is just to get your blood flowing to warm up muscles, tendons, and joints.

> **5-FACTOR HOLLYWOOD WORKOUT**
> Phase 1: Cardio Warm-up
> Phase 2: Upper-Body Strength Training
> Phase 3: Lower-Body Strength Training
> Phase 4: Core Training
> Phase 5: Cardio Work

Begin at a low intensity. Gradually increase the intensity by speeding up the activity you're doing. By the end of the 5 minutes, I want your heart rate elevated so you're in a fat-burning zone when you start Phases 2 and 3.

As you warm up, check your pulse by placing two fingers either on the side of your neck or on the front of your wrist just below your palm. Count the heartbeats for 10 seconds, then multiply that number by 6 to determine your pulse rate in beats per minute (BPM). By the end of your warm-up, your BPM should fall within the appropriate range below to burn fat efficiently. (If your BPM is less than suggested, up your intensity in the next workout; if it's higher than suggested, lower your intensity in the next workout.)

Age	Pulse	Age	Pulse
20–24	130–170	55–59	107–140
25–29	127–166	60–64	104–136
30–34	124–162	65–69	101–132
35–39	120–157	70–74	98–128
40–44	117–153	75–79	94–123
45–49	114–149	80+	91–119
50–54	111–145		

PHASES 2 AND 3: 10 MINUTES OF STRENGTH TRAINING (UPPER AND LOWER BODY)

Phase 2 and Phase 3, which together work all of the upper- and lower-body muscles, are combined for a good reason—to keep your heart rate elevated so you burn fat as you build muscle.

For 10 minutes, you'll do two different exercises back-to-back, resting only after completing a superset made up of both exercises. Refer to the charts below to see how many repetitions to perform (it varies by week) and how many seconds to rest between supersets. Repeat this cycle for the prescribed number of supersets.

Here are the 10 exercises you'll use over the course of the week.

Day	Exercise	Core muscles involved
1: Monday	Incline Dumbbell Flys (upper body)	Chest
	Ball Wall Squats (lower body)	Quadriceps
2: Tuesday	Reverse Incline Dumbbell Rows (upper body)	Back
	Dumbbell Deadlifts (lower body)	Hamstrings
3: Wednesday	Off	
4: Thursday	Incline Dumbbell Bicep Curls (upper body)	Biceps
	Overhead Dumbbell Tricep Extensions (upper body)	Triceps
5: Friday	Dumbbell Lateral Raises (upper body)	Shoulders
	Step-Ups (lower body)	Quadriceps
6: Saturday	Bent-Over Dumbbell Rows (upper body)	Back
	Lying Ball Hamstring Curls (lower body)	Hamstrings
7: Sunday	Off	

If you're a beginner or intermediate exerciser, here's your plan!

Week	For each exercise	Rest after each superset
1	25 reps, 2 supersets,	80 seconds
2	20 reps, 3 supersets	70 seconds
3	15 reps, 3 supersets	60 seconds
4	16 reps, 4 supersets	50 seconds
5	10 reps, 5 supersets	40 seconds

If you're an advanced exerciser, here's your plan!

Week	For each exercise	Rest after each superset
1	30 reps, 3 supersets	90 seconds
2	25 reps, 3 supersets	70 seconds
3	20 reps, 4 supersets	50 seconds
4	15 reps, 4 supersets	40 seconds
5	12 reps, 5 supersets	30 seconds

As you see, you'll be varying the repetitions and adding more supersets as the weeks progress. The rest time between supersets also decreases each week. The exercises themselves stay the same throughout this 5-week plan.

THE ONLY EQUIPMENT YOU NEED

To do the 5-Factor Workout, all you need is a set of dumbbells, a bench with an incline feature (if you don't have one, modify the exercises as described), and a stability ball.

When using dumbbells, pick a weight that's heavy enough so you can just barely complete the prescribed repetitions with perfect form. For example, if an exercise calls for you to do 16 repetitions and you could have done 18, your dumbbell isn't heavy enough to work your muscles, and you're cheating yourself of results.

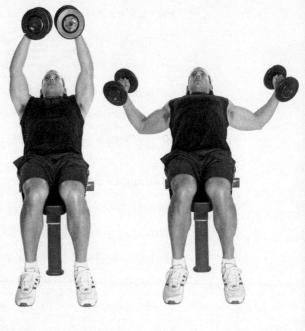

STRENGTH TRAINING EXERCISES
DAY 1: MONDAY

INCLINE DUMBBELL FLYS

Lie flat on your back on an incline bench with a dumbbell in each hand. Raise your arms above you so the weights come together directly above your chest, palms facing each other. Bend your elbows slightly and slowly lower your arms out to the sides until the weights are in line with your chest. Slowly sweep your arms back up until they are over your chest—imagine you're hugging a wide barrel—and repeat.

If you don't have an incline bench: Do this exercise while lying on a flat bench instead.

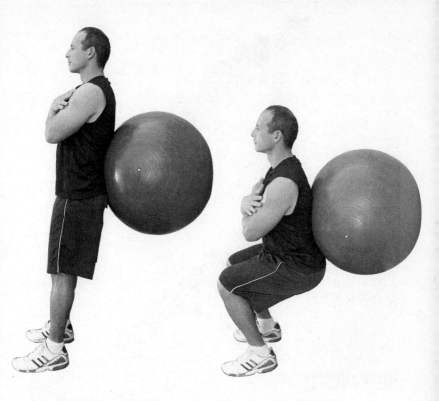

BALL WALL SQUATS

Stand a few feet away from a wall with your back toward the wall. Tuck a
stability ball between your back and the wall, then lean back against the
ball until your entire upper body is supported by the ball and the wall.
Maintaining your balance, cross your arms in front of your chest, then slowly
squat down until your thighs are parallel to the floor. The ball should roll
down the wall as you go. Slowly stand back up and repeat.

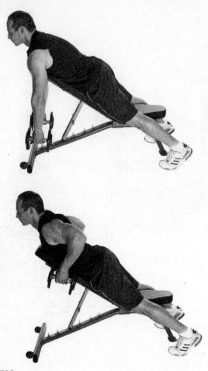

DAY 2: TUESDAY

REVERSE INCLINE DUMBBELL ROWS

Lie facedown on an incline bench, with your chest flat against the elevated pad. Hold a dumbbell in each hand, letting your arms hang down to the floor, palms facing each other. Keeping your chest on the bench and your arms close to your torso, pull both dumbbells up to the sides of your chest. Slowly lower your arms back down and repeat.

If you don't have an incline bench: You can do the exercise one arm at a time. Stand with your right side toward a bench—or bed—and a dumbbell in your left hand. Rest your right hand and knee on the bench, bend forward at the waist, and let your left arm hang down toward the floor. Slowly pull the weight up to the side of your chest, then lower it. Repeat with other arm.

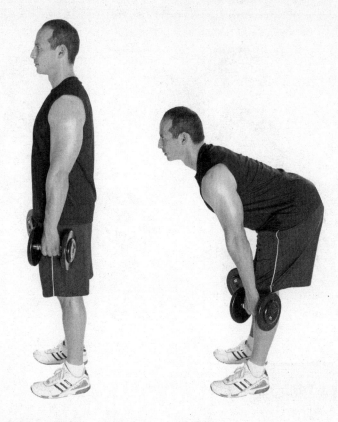

DUMBBELL DEADLIFTS

Position a dumbbell on the floor along the outside of each foot, then stand tall. Bend your knees and grasp the dumbbells with your palms facing in. Keeping your head up and your back straight, slowly stand up until your legs are straight, knees unlocked. Make sure the weights stay close to your body as you stand. Slowly reverse the motion and place the dumbbells back down on the floor. Repeat.

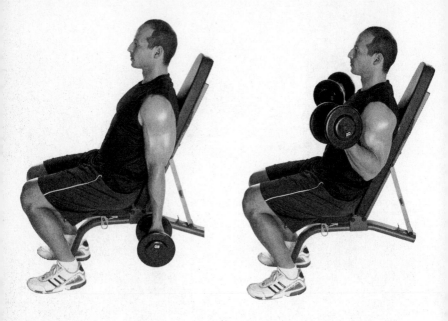

DAY 4: THURSDAY

INCLINE DUMBBELL BICEP CURLS

Lie faceup on an incline bench with a dumbbell in each hand, letting your
arms hang straight down toward the floor. Your palms should face up toward
the front. Keeping your upper arms stationary, slowly curl both weights up
until they are in front of your chest—remember to curl both weights up at
the same time. Slowly lower the weights back down and repeat.

If you don't have an incline bench: Do this exercise standing up instead.

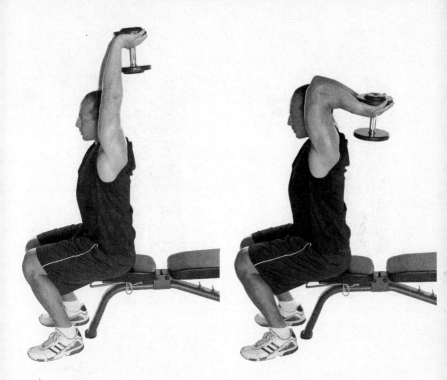

OVERHEAD DUMBBELL TRICEP EXTENSIONS

Sit on a chair or an exercise bench with your back straight. Place your feet firmly on the floor and grasp a single dumbbell with both hands. Raise the weight above your head, rotating it so the top plate rests comfortably in the palms of your hands, with your thumbs around the handle. Slowly lower the weight behind your head until your forearms touch your biceps. Straighten your arms to raise the weight back over your head. Repeat.

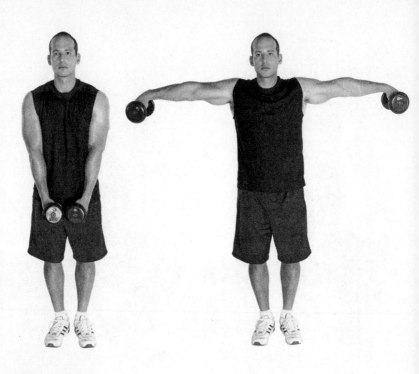

DAY 5: FRIDAY

DUMBBELL LATERAL RAISES

Stand with your arms in front of you with a dumbbell in each hand, palms facing each other. Keeping your arms straight and your wrists slightly bent, slowly raise the weights out to the sides until your arms are parallel to the floor (you'll look like the letter T). Pause for a second, then slowly lower your arms back down in front of you so the dumbbells touch each other right below your waistline. Repeat.

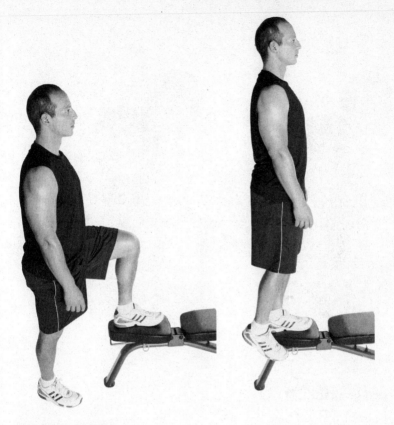

STEP-UPS

Stand in front of an exercise bench (or a sturdy box or staircase). Let your arms hang at your sides. With your back straight, place your left foot on the bench and push yourself up onto the bench until your left leg is straight. You don't have to bring your right foot onto the bench unless you need to balance yourself. Reverse the exercise by stepping back down and placing both feet back on the floor. Repeat the exercise, using the same leg, for the number of repetitions prescribed. Then change positions to work the opposite leg, this time placing your right foot on the bench.

For added intensity, you may do this exercise while holding a dumbbell in each hand.

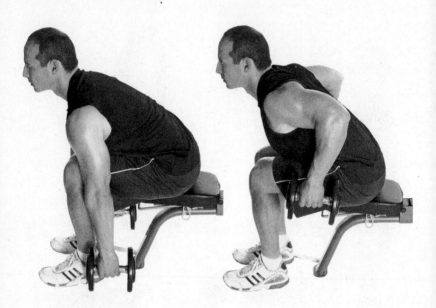

DAY 6: SATURDAY

BENT-OVER DUMBBELL ROWS

Sit on the edge of a bench holding a dumbbell in each hand. Bend forward at the waist—keeping your back flat—until your back is almost parallel to the floor (your chest should come down as close to your thighs as possible). Let your arms hang straight down, with palms facing each other. Slowly draw your elbows up as high as you can, keeping your arms close to your sides. Pause, then slowly lower them back down until your arms are straight once again. Repeat.

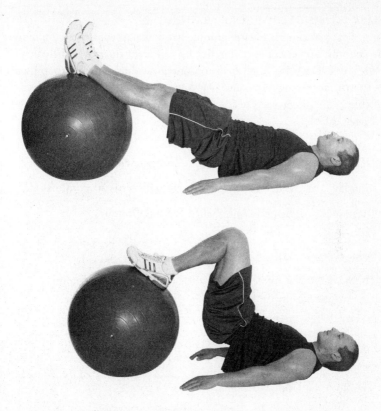

LYING BALL HAMSTRING CURLS

Lie flat on your back with your arms flat on the floor and your heels on top of a stability ball. Press your heels down onto the ball, then tighten your core muscles. Slowly raise your hips up and draw your heels—and the ball—toward your butt as far as you can. Pause, then roll the ball back by straightening your legs; your hips will naturally lower back to the floor as you reverse the motion. Repeat.

PHASE 4: 5 MINUTES OF CORE TRAINING

Phase 4 targets all four muscle groups that make up your core. You'll do one abdominal exercise each day, but five different ones over the course of the week. Days 1–4 each focus on one individual muscle group plus the specific ab-toning move, and Day 5 works as many muscle groups as possible in one single exercise.

Here's the plan:

Day	Exercise	Core muscles involved
1: Monday	Ball Crunches	Upper Rectus Abdominis
2: Tuesday	Seated Dumbbell Side Bends	Lateral Obliques
3: Wednesday	Off	
4: Thursday	Reverse Ball Crunches	Lower Rectus Abdominis
5: Friday	Ball Twists	Transversus Abdominis
6: Saturday	Ball Tuck Crunches	Upper/Lower Rectus Abdominis
7: Sunday	Off	

If you're a beginner or intermediate exerciser, here's your plan!

Week	For each exercise	Rest after each superset
1	3 sets, 10 reps	15 seconds
2	3 sets, 15 reps	20 seconds
3	3 sets, 20 reps	25 seconds
4	3 sets, 25 reps	30 seconds
5	3 sets, 30 reps	35 seconds

If you're an advanced exerciser, here's your plan!

Week	For each exercise	Rest after each superset
1	4 sets, 20 reps	10 seconds
2	4 sets, 25 reps	15 seconds
3	4 sets, 30 reps	20 seconds
4	4 sets, 35 reps	25 seconds
5	4 sets, 40 reps	30 seconds

You'll be doing more repetitions as the weeks go on. The rest time between sets also increases each week. The 5 core exercises—just like the exercises in Phases 2 and 3—will stay the same throughout the entire 5-week plan.

> **I wanted to lose pregnancy weight, plus get in shape for health reasons. But I was getting tired of working out and never seeing results. I was never a couch potato, so I became frustrated when I wasn't seeing any change in my body. 5-Factor changed that. I started to finally see muscle definition, and I love how little time it takes to complete a workout.**
>
> **Holly Flom** AGE: **37** WEIGHT LOST SO FAR: **29 lbs.**

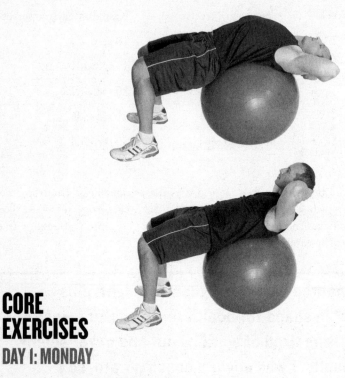

CORE EXERCISES
DAY 1: MONDAY

BALL CRUNCHES

Sit on a stability ball with your feet flat on the floor. Place your hands along the sides of your head. Keeping your feet flat on the floor, slowly lean back until your head, shoulders, and back are all touching the ball. This is the starting position. Slowly curl your shoulders and upper back up off the ball. Lower yourself back down on the ball and repeat.

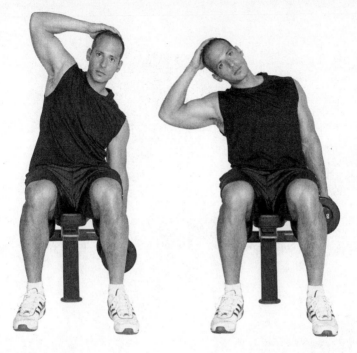

DAY 2: TUESDAY

SEATED DUMBBELL SIDE BENDS

Sit on a chair or bench, holding a dumbbell in your left hand, palm facing in. Rest your right hand on the top of your head and let your left arm hang straight down along your side. Keeping your left arm straight, take a breath and bend at the waist to the right as far as you comfortably can. Return to the starting position, then bend at the waist to the left. Return to the starting position and repeat the exercise for the prescribed number of repetitions. Then switch positions, placing the weight in your right hand and your left hand on top of your head, and repeat the exercise.

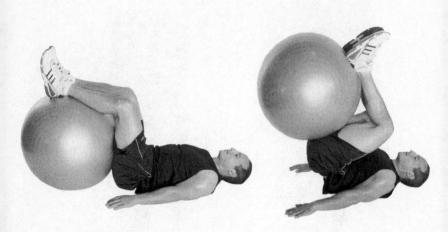

DAY 4: THURSDAY

REVERSE BALL CRUNCH

Lie flat on the floor faceup and with your knees bent. Place a stability ball behind your knees and draw your feet toward your butt to tuck the ball in place. Extend your arms straight down at your sides, with your palms pressed flat on the floor. This is the start position. Keeping the ball tucked underneath your legs, slowly curl your knees toward your chest. Pause, lower your legs back down until the ball touches the floor, and repeat.

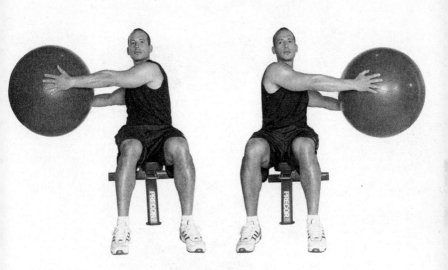

DAY 5: FRIDAY

BALL TWISTS

Sit on a bench with your knees bent and your feet flat on the floor. Hold
a stability ball with both hands and extend your arms above your chest.
Keeping your arms straight, twist to the right. Bring the ball back to the front
so it's directly in front of you. Then repeat the move, this time twisting to the
left. Alternate right and left throughout the set.

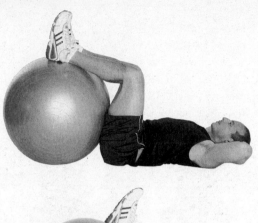

DAY 6: SATURDAY

BALL TUCK CRUNCH

Position yourself as if you were going to do a sit-up, but instead of keeping your feet on the floor, place them up on a stability ball. Your heels should press against the top of the ball. Keeping your arms bent behind your head, lift your hips and draw your knees toward your midsection—the ball should naturally roll toward your head. Hold, then extend your legs back until they're back in the starting position. Repeat.

PHASE 5: 5 MINUTES (OR LONGER) OF CARDIO WORK

For the last phase, go back to whatever activity you were doing in Phase 1. This time, it should feel easy to work at the same high intensity you achieved at the end of Phase 1. Start exercising, bring your pulse rate back up to your target BPM, and maintain that pace for 5 minutes. If you can go longer and have the time, go for it. The longer you can exercise, the more calories you'll burn overall. Personally, I would go for no more than 10 minutes total so I'd have enough energy for the next day's workout.

SUMMARY OF THE 5-FACTOR HOLLYWOOD WORKOUT

PHASE 1

Five minutes of cardio warm-up

PHASES 2 AND 3

Ten minutes of strength training

Day	Exercise	Core muscles involved
1: Monday	Incline Dumbbell Flys Ball Wall Squats	Chest Quadriceps
2: Tuesday	Reverse Incline Dumbbell Rows Dumbbell Deadlifts	Back Hamstrings
3: Wednesday	Off	
4: Thursday	Incline Dumbbell Bicep Curls Overhead Dumbbell Triceps Extensions	Biceps Triceps
5: Friday	Dumbbell Lateral Raises Step-Ups	Shoulders Quadriceps
6: Saturday	Bent-Over Dumbbell Rows Lying Ball Hamstring Curls	Back Hamstrings
7: Sunday	Off	

PHASE 4
Five minutes of core training

Day	Exercise	Core muscles involved
1: Monday	Ball Crunches	Upper Rectus Abdominis
2: Tuesday	Seated Dumbbell Side Bends	Lateral Obliques
3: Wednesday	Off	
4: Thursday	Reverse Ball Crunches	Lower Rectus Abdominis
5: Friday	Ball Twists	Transversus Abdominis
6: Saturday	Ball Tuck Crunches	Upper/Lower Rectus Abdominis
7: Sunday	Off	

PHASE 5
Five minutes of cardio work

THE 5-MONTH 5-FACTOR CHALLENGE

After you complete the 5-week 5-Factor program, you can repeat it for as long as you like. Its built-in variety makes it a constant challenge for your muscles, so they continue to reap the benefits with each and every cycle. If you're up for a new challenge, I've designed a 5-month plan that really keeps your body guessing—and the results coming!

Follow the same exercises in this chapter and do the required reps, sets, and rest intervals I've indicated in the chart on page 109. In the middle of the plan, you'll take a break from the strength training and core exercises by doing cardio for 25 minutes for all 5 workouts for a week. Are you up for my 5-Factor fitness challenge? Ready, set, go!

If you're an advanced exerciser, here's your plan!

Week	For each exercise	Rest after each superset
1	16 reps, 3 supersets	60 seconds
2	12 reps, 3 supersets	55 seconds
3	10 reps, 4 supersets	50 seconds
4	12 reps, 3 supersets	55 seconds
5	16 reps, 3 supersets	60 seconds
6	20 reps, 3 supersets	60 seconds
7	16 reps, 3 supersets	55 seconds
8	12 reps, 4 supersets	50 seconds
9	10 reps, 4 supersets	45 seconds
10	16 reps, 4 supersets	50 seconds
11	20 reps, 3 supersets	55 seconds
Cardio	25 minutes	
12	25 reps, 3 supersets	60 seconds
13	20 reps, 4 supersets	55 seconds
14	16 reps, 4 supersets	50 seconds
15	12 reps, 5 supersets	45 seconds
16	10 reps, 5 supersets	40 seconds
17	12 reps, 5 supersets	45 seconds
18	16 reps, 4 supersets	50 seconds
19	20 reps, 4 supersets	55 seconds
20	25 reps, 3 supersets	60 seconds

CHAPTER 10

5-Factor
Recipes

Most diet books tell you exactly what meals to eat and in what order. Who eats like that? I don't, and I know you don't either.

At the end of this book, I'll make suggestions for arranging my 120 5-Factor recipes into a weeklong plan. But whether you eat them in the recommended order is entirely up to you.

I want you to be creative. That's what makes the 5-Factor Diet so effective—and easy to stick to. Use these menus in whichever order keeps you coming back for more. When I work with Kanye West, for instance, he likes to eat the same thing for breakfast on most days: an egg white omelet with a little lean shredded beef and a bowl of berries. His favorite breakfast helps him stick to eating healthy.

Alicia Keys, on the other hand, loves to cook, and that gives her the ability to be more experimental. She enjoys variety in her diet and loves to try different 5-Factor menus.

If you want to eat the same breakfast every single morning, I have no problem with that. And if you prefer to mix things up every day, that's fine too. Each of the 120 recipes in this book is balanced nutritionally and specifically to meet the 5-Factor criteria. That way, even if you chose to eat the same five meals every day—or even the same meal five times a day!—you'd never be left nutrient-deficient.

I'm presenting you with 120 recipes—nearly a month's worth of meals—because variety is important to many dieters. These 120 fantastic recipes—just like the 100 recipes in *5-Factor Fitness*—not only are delicious but also are hands-down some of the easiest and most convenient recipes you'll ever try. I should know because I've had to make them on the fly for my clients at the strangest places and times.

FAST, FUN, AND DELICIOUS

When I'm on film sets with clients, I prepare their food quite often. I literally have minutes to make a meal when they unexpectedly take a break from filming. It was that kind of pressure that inspired my recipes.

Each had to be very simple to make.

Each had to use very few ingredients.

Each had to be delicious—I'm competing against catered food on sets, you know! (Halle Berry loves my 5-Factor fajitas, while Eva Mendes flips over my 5-Factor pizzas.)

And finally, each had to meet my 5-Factor criteria.

That's exactly what these recipes deliver. Not only do they fulfill the 5-Factor criteria, but they can be prepared—minus cook time—in just five minutes. You need only five—or fewer—core ingredients (plus seasonings and oils). I kept the number of steps in each recipe to five as well. If you want even more variety, I encourage you to check out the recipes in *5-Factor Fitness*.

It's easy to make 5-Factor meals and enjoy the benefits of the 5-Factor Diet. So let's get cooking!

No more excuses.

Meal 1. Breakfast

Asparagus Crepes with Toast

1 bunch asparagus spears

1½ cups egg whites

⅔ cup nonfat milk

4 slices whole grain bread, toasted

Salt and cracked black pepper to taste

Cooking oil spray

1. Place the asparagus spears in a container with a little water. Microwave for 1½ minutes, then drain and set aside.

2. Whisk together the egg whites, milk, salt, and pepper.

3. Coat a nonstick skillet with cooking spray and heat the skillet. Pour half of the egg whites into the skillet. When the egg whites begin to set, turn them over. Cook for 30 seconds and then slide the crepe onto a cutting board. Place half of the asparagus spears in the center of the crepe and roll tightly. Repeat but reserve a couple of asparagus spears for garnish.

To Serve: Place the asparagus crepes on plates and serve with toast. Garnish with the reserved asparagus spears.

Servings: 2

Frittata Italiana

1. Whisk together the egg whites, cream cheese, salt, and pepper.

2. Spray a nonstick skillet with cooking spray and heat the skillet. Add the egg white mixture and cook until it begins to set. Immediately add the sun-dried tomatoes and basil leaves. Cover and cook about 2 minutes or until the eggs are completely set.

To Serve: Slide the frittata onto a cutting board and cut into four wedges. Serve two wedges and two slices of toast on each plate. Garnish with pepper and additional fresh basil.

Servings: 2

1½ cups egg whites

¼ cup nonfat cream cheese, softened

1 cup finely chopped sun-dried tomatoes

4 leaves fresh basil, finely chopped

4 slices whole grain bread, toasted

Salt and cracked black pepper to taste

Cooking oil spray

Breakfast Burritos I

¾ cup egg whites

2 whole grain or whole wheat tortillas

2¼ cups canned black beans, drained

½ cup shredded nonfat mozzarella cheese

I cup salsa

I teaspoon ground cumin

I teaspoon garlic salt

Cracked black pepper to taste

Cooking oil spray

1. Preheat the oven or toaster oven to 350°F.

2. Whisk together the egg whites, cumin, garlic salt, and pepper. Coat a nonstick skillet with cooking spray and heat the skillet. Add the egg white mixture. Cook and stir over low heat until egg whites are cooked. Set aside.

3. Lay tortillas on a cutting board and sprinkle with black beans. Top with the egg whites and shredded cheese and roll tightly. Wrap the burritos in foil and bake for 2 minutes.

To Serve: Unwrap the burritos, cut in half, and serve with salsa.

Servings: 2

Breakfast Burritos II

1. Whisk together the ricotta cheese, egg whites, taco seasoning mix, onion powder, salt, and pepper. Stir in the tomatoes. Coat a nonstick skillet with cooking spray and heat the skillet. Add the egg mixture. Cook and stir until the egg whites are cooked. Set aside.

2. Heat the tortillas in the microwave for 20 seconds and place on a cutting board. Place the scrambled eggs and spinach in the center of each tortilla. Roll tightly.

To Serve: Cut the burritos in half and serve hot.

Servings: 2

1 cup nonfat ricotta cheese

¼ cup egg whites

4 cups diced tomatoes

4 whole grain or whole wheat tortillas

8 cups spinach leaves

2 teaspoons taco seasoning mix

1 teaspoon onion powder

Salt and cracked black pepper to taste

Cooking oil spray

Breakfast Burritos III

2 cups egg whites

2 large whole grain or whole wheat tortillas

1¼ cups refried beans

¼ cup shredded nonfat cheddar cheese

1 cup salsa

Cooking oil spray

1. Coat a nonstick skillet with cooking spray and heat the skillet. Add the egg whites. Cook and stir for 1½ minutes. Set aside.

2. Heat the tortillas in the microwave for 15 seconds. Spread the tortillas with refried beans and spoon the egg whites over the beans. Sprinkle with cheese and roll the tortillas tightly.

To Serve: Cut the burritos in half and serve with salsa.

Servings: 2

Broccoli-Cheddar Omelet

1. Whisk together the egg whites, Mrs. Dash, salt, and pepper. Coat a nonstick skillet with cooking spray and heat the skillet. Add the broccoli florets and cook and stir until they are bright green. Add the egg whites and cook while gently pushing them to the center with a rubber spatula. When the egg mixture begins to set on the bottom, turn it over. Sprinkle with cheese and cover the pan. Cook for 30 seconds or until the cheese begins to melt.

To Serve: Slide the omelet onto a plate and fold in half. Cut in half and serve with toast.

Servings: 2

NOTE: You can use any green vegetable in your refrigerator in place of the broccoli.

1¼ cups egg whites

3 cups broccoli florets, coarsely chopped

¼ cup shredded nonfat cheddar cheese

4 slices whole grain bread, toasted

1 teaspoon Mrs. Dash seasoning mix

Salt and cracked black pepper to taste

Cooking oil spray

Bell Pepper Pancakes with Mozzarella and Crisp Bacon

1½ cups egg whites

2¾ cups diced bell peppers

1 tablespoon nonfat sour cream

¼ cup shredded nonfat mozzarella cheese

2 strips turkey bacon

Salt and cracked black pepper to taste

Cooking oil spray

1. Preheat broiler. Whisk together the egg whites, bell peppers, sour cream, salt, and pepper.

2. Coat a nonstick crepe pan with cooking spray and heat the pan. Ladle ¼ cup of the egg white mixture into the pan and cook until it is partially set. Turn it over and cook until almost set. Repeat with the remaining egg white mixture. Place the pancakes on a nonstick baking sheet and sprinkle with the mozzarella cheese. Broil until the cheese is melted and golden brown.

3. Microwave the turkey bacon for 3 minutes.

To Serve: Transfer the pancakes and turkey bacon to serving plates.

Servings: 2

The Cowboy Omelet

1. Microwave the sweet potatoes for 3 minutes each. Peel the potatoes and set aside.

2. Whisk together the egg whites, chili powder, garlic powder, salt, and pepper. Coat a nonstick skillet with cooking spray and heat the skillet. Add the mushrooms and cook until most of the liquid has evaporated. Add the egg white mixture and cook until it begins to set. Add the Canadian bacon and cheddar cheese. Cover and cook until the cheese is melted.

To Serve: Cut the sweet potatoes into cubes and gently toss with the cinnamon, salt, and pepper. Cut the omelet in half and serve with the sweet potatoes.

Servings: 2

2 medium sweet potatoes

1 cup egg whites

5 cups sliced button mushrooms

1 ounce Canadian bacon, cut into thin strips

1 cup shredded nonfat cheddar cheese

1 teaspoon chili powder

½ teaspoon garlic powder

Salt and cracked black pepper to taste

Cooking oil spray

1 pinch ground cinnamon

Egg and Veggie Muffins

1⅛ cups egg whites

1¾ cups broccoli florets, coarsely chopped

¾ cup diced red and green bell pepper

½ cup shredded nonfat mozzarella cheese

4 slices whole grain bread, toasted

Salt and cracked black pepper to taste

Cooking oil spray

1. Preheat the oven to 350°F.

2. Whisk together the egg whites, salt, and pepper. Coat 12 muffin cups with cooking spray. Pour the eggs into the muffin cups, filling each cup halfway. Drop the broccoli and bell pepper into the egg whites, dividing them evenly. Bake for 10 minutes or until the egg begins to set. Remove from the oven and sprinkle cheese over the top of each muffin. Return to the oven and bake until the egg has set completely and the cheese is melted and golden.

To Serve: Slide a knife around the edge of each muffin and unmold onto a cutting board. Cut in half or leave whole. Place on plates and serve with toast.

Servings: 2

Open-Face Egg and Bacon Sandwiches

1. Microwave the turkey bacon strips for 3 minutes or until crisp. Set aside.

2. Whisk together the egg whites, salt, and pepper. Coat a nonstick skillet with cooking spray and heat the skillet. Add the egg white mixture. Cook and stir about 1½ minutes or until the egg whites are set.

To Serve: Spoon the egg whites on the toast. Top with cheese, turkey bacon, and diced tomatoes.

Servings: 2

NOTE: If you can't find nonfat cheddar cheese, you can substitute shredded part-skim mozzarella cheese.

2 strips turkey bacon

1¼ cups egg whites

4 slices whole grain bread, toasted

½ cup shredded nonfat cheddar cheese

1¼ cups diced, seeded plum tomatoes

Salt and cracked black pepper to taste

Cooking oil spray

Red Bell Pepper Frittata with Baked Yams

2 cups egg whites

1½ cups coarsely chopped roasted
red peppers

1 cup shredded nonfat mozzarella cheese

2 large yams

2 teaspoons onion powder

1 teaspoon ground cumin

Salt and cracked black pepper to taste

Cooking oil spray

1. Whisk together the egg whites, onion powder, cumin, salt, and black pepper. Stir in the roasted peppers and shredded cheese. Coat a small glass baking dish with cooking spray. Pour the egg white mixture into the baking dish. Microwave for 4 minutes. Set aside. Microwave the yams for 3½ minutes each. Cut the yams in half and season with salt and pepper.

To Serve: Cut the frittata and serve with yams. Garnish with cracked black pepper.

Servings: 2

Salmon-Leek Frittata with Whole Grain Toast

1. Whisk together the egg whites, leeks, salt, and pepper. Coat a small glass baking dish with cooking spray. Pour the egg white mixture into the baking dish. Cover with plastic wrap three-fourths of the way. Microwave for 4 minutes. Cool for 3 minutes.

To Serve: Run a knife around the edge of the frittata and turn it over onto a cutting board. Spread the frittata with cream cheese and top with chopped salmon. Cut frittata in half and serve with toast. Garnish with parsley and additional pepper.

Servings: 2

1½ cups egg whites

1 cup sliced leeks (white part only)

2 tablespoons nonfat cream cheese

2 ounces smoked salmon, chopped

4 slices whole grain bread, toasted

Salt and cracked black pepper

Cooking oil spray

2 teaspoons dried parsley

Scrambled Egg Casserole

1 plum tomato, seeded and diced

1 tablespoon thinly sliced scallion, white part only

¾ cup egg whites

½ cup shredded nonfat mozzarella cheese

4 slices whole grain bread, toasted

Cooking oil spray

Salt and cracked black pepper to taste

1. Coat a nonstick skillet with cooking spray and heat the skillet. Add the tomato and scallion and cook until the scallion is light golden. Whisk in the egg whites and half of the shredded cheese. Cook and stir until the egg white mixture is almost set. Season with salt and pepper.

To Serve: Spoon the scrambled eggs into a small casserole and sprinkle with the remaining cheese. Microwave until the cheese is melted. Serve with toast.

Servings: 2

Scrambled Eggs with Toast and Grapefruit

1. Coat a nonstick skillet with cooking spray and heat the skillet. Add the cubed chicken and egg whites. Season with salt and pepper and cook for 2 minutes. Add the cheese and cook until the cheese is melted.

To Serve: Spoon the scrambled eggs onto plates and serve with toast and grapefruit.

Servings: 2

¼ pound smoked chicken breast, cut into cubes

¼ cup egg whites

½ cup shredded nonfat cheddar cheese

4 slices whole grain bread, toasted

2 grapefruit, cut in half and seeded

Cooking oil spray

Salt and cracked black pepper to taste

Smoked Salmon Omelet with Cream Cheese and Whole Grain Toast

1 cup egg whites

¼ cup nonfat cream cheese, softened

2 ounces smoked salmon

4 slices whole grain bread, toasted

1¾ cups orange sections

Salt and cracked black pepper to taste

Cooking oil spray

1. Whisk together the egg whites, cream cheese, salt, and pepper. Coat a nonstick skillet with cooking spray and heat the skillet. Pour the egg white mixture into the skillet. Gently push the egg whites toward the center as they cook. When they are almost set, place the smoked salmon on top. Cover the pan and cook for 30 seconds. Remove the lid and season with additional pepper.

To serve: Slide the omelet onto a cutting board and fold in half. Cut the omelet in half and serve with toast and orange segments.

Servings: 2

Smoked Turkey and Tomato Scrambled Eggs with Toast

1. Coat a nonstick skillet with cooking spray and heat the skillet. Add the egg whites and cook for 30 seconds. Sprinkle with chopped turkey, tomatoes, and shredded cheese. Cook and stir about 2 minutes or until the egg whites are completely set. Season with salt and pepper.

To Serve: Serve the scrambled eggs with toast.

Servings: 2

NOTE: For lunch, spoon the scrambled eggs on toast and eat it as an open-face sandwich.

I cup egg whites

3 ounces deli-style fat-free smoked turkey, chopped

1½ cups chopped plum tomatoes

½ cup shredded nonfat mozzarella cheese

4 slices whole grain bread, toasted

Cooking oil spray

Salt and cracked black pepper to taste

Sweet Potato Home Fries and Scrambled Eggs

2 large sweet potatoes

½ cup diced Spanish onion

I bell pepper, seeded and diced

I cup egg whites

I cup shredded nonfat cheddar cheese

Cooking oil spray

1½ teaspoons garlic powder

I teaspoon paprika

I teaspoon red pepper flakes

Salt and cracked black pepper to taste

1. Microwave the sweet potatoes for 3½ minutes each or until tender. Peel off the skins and dice the potatoes. Coat a nonstick skillet with cooking spray and heat the skillet. Add the onion and cook for 1 minute. Add the sweet potatoes, bell pepper, garlic powder, paprika, and red pepper flakes. Toss gently and set aside.

2. Coat a nonstick skillet with cooking spray and heat the skillet. Add the egg whites, cheese, salt, and cracked black pepper. Cook and stir until the egg whites are set.

To Serve: Spoon the scrambled eggs and home fries onto plates. Garnish with cracked black pepper.

Servings: 2

NOTE: If you can't find nonfat cheddar cheese, use shredded part-skim mozzarella.

Ham Steaks with Applesauce and Toast

1. Place the ham steaks in a hot nonstick skillet and cook for 1 minute on each side. In a bowl, toss together the apple pieces, cinnamon, and sugar substitute. Microwave for 2 minutes. Mash the cooked apples and the cottage cheese with a fork.

To Serve: Serve ham steaks with applesauce and toast.

Servings: 2

⅓ pound extra lean ham, cut into two serving-size pieces

2¾ cups peeled, cored, and cut-up Fuji apples

½ cup nonfat cottage cheese

2 slices whole grain bread, toasted

1 teaspoon ground cinnamon

¼ teaspoon sugar substitute

Bran Pancakes with Ricotta

½ cup bran flakes

½ cup egg whites

½ cup nonfat sour cream

1¾ cups nonfat ricotta cheese

1 tablespoon sugar substitute

1 pinch salt

Butter-flavor cooking oil spray

2 teaspoons ground cinnamon

1. Whisk together the bran flakes, egg whites, sour cream, sugar substitute, and salt. Coat a nonstick skillet with cooking spray and heat the skillet. Ladle a thin layer of batter into the skillet. Cook until the batter begins to set. Carefully turn the pancake and cook on the other side until the pancake is completely set and is a light golden color. Repeat with the remaining batter.

To Serve: Dust the pancakes with cinnamon and serve with ricotta.

Servings: 2

Oatmeal-Berry Pancakes

1. Beat together the egg whites, strawberries, rolled oats, and sugar substitute until smooth.

2. Coat a nonstick skillet with cooking spray and heat the skillet. Ladle ¼ cup of the batter into the skillet. Cook until the batter is set around the edges of the pan, then push it toward the center with a spatula. Cook until the batter begins to set in the center. Turn the pancake over or cover the pan. Cook for 1 minute. Repeat with remaining batter.

To Serve: Slide the pancakes onto plates and top with sour cream. Garnish with blueberries.

Servings: 2

1½ cups egg whites

1⅓ cups chopped strawberries

1 cup rolled oats

1 cup nonfat sour cream

1 cup blueberries

1¼ teaspoons sugar substitute

Butter-flavor cooking oil spray

French Toast with Ricotta

⅔ cup egg whites

⅔ cup nonfat milk

2 slices whole grain bread

⅛ cup nonfat ricotta cheese

1 teaspoon sugar substitute

1 pinch salt

Cooking oil spray

1 teaspoon ground cinnamon

1. Whisk together the egg whites, milk, sugar substitute, and salt. Soak the bread in the egg white mixture. Drain the excess liquid.

2. Coat a nonstick skillet with cooking spay and heat the skillet. Cook the bread, one slice at a time, until each side is set and bread is light brown.

To Serve: Place the French toast on a plate and top with ricotta. Garnish with cinnamon.

Servings: 1

Fully Charged Fruit Salad

1. Peel and section three of the oranges and squeeze the juice from the fourth orange. Whisk the orange juice, protein powder, and ginger into the cottage cheese.

To Serve: Spoon the cottage cheese into bowls and top with orange sections, apple wedges, and strawberries. Serve chilled.

Servings: 2

4 oranges

I scoop protein powder (100% whey)

I cup nonfat cottage cheese

2 Granny Smith apples, cored and cut into wedges

2 cups quartered strawberries

I teaspoon ground ginger

Cream of Wheat and Protein

2¼ cups nonfat milk

¾ cup Cream of Wheat

I scoop protein powder (100% whey)

I teaspoon ground cinnamon

1. In a saucepan, combine the milk, Cream of Wheat, and protein powder and bring to a boil. Whisk until smooth and creamy.

To Serve: Ladle into bowls and garnish with cinnamon.

Servings: 2

NOTE: If you can't find 100% whey protein, use soy protein.

Kashi GoLean with Nonfat Milk

To Serve: Place 1 cup of cereal in each bowl and add the milk.

Servings: 2

NOTE: You can find Kashi GoLean cereal in the organic section of your local market.

2 cups Kashi GoLean cereal or other high-fiber whole grain cereal

2 cups nonfat milk

Meals 2 and 4. Snacks

Apple-Turkey Roll-Ups with Relish and Mustard

5 ounces deli-style turkey breast, sliced

3 Granny Smith apples, cored and thinly sliced

2 tablespoons pickle relish

I tablespoon whole grain mustard

1. Place the turkey slices on a cutting board. Lay the apple slices on the turkey and spread with relish and mustard. Roll tightly and secure each with a toothpick.

To Serve: Make the roll-ups ahead, wrap in plastic wrap, and refrigerate.

Servings: 2

Belgian Endive Stuffed with Cheesy Artichoke Spread

1. In a food processor, pulse the artichoke hearts, cream cheese, mozzarella cheese, parsley, onion powder, salt, and pepper.

To Serve: Pull the leaves from the endive and arrange them on a serving platter. Spoon the artichoke spread into the leaves.

Servings: 2

2 cups canned artichoke hearts, drained

½ cup nonfat cream cheese, softened

2 tablespoons shredded nonfat mozzarella cheese

1 whole Belgian endive

1 teaspoon dried parsley

1 teaspoon onion powder

Salt and cracked black pepper to taste

Bruschetta

¾ cup finely chopped sun-dried tomatoes

4 whole grain crackers

⅔ cup shredded nonfat mozzarella cheese

1 teaspoon garlic powder

½ teaspoon onion powder

1 teaspoon Italian seasoning

Cracked black pepper to taste

1. Preheat broiler to medium. Spoon the sun-dried tomatoes onto the crackers and top with the mozzarella cheese. Season with garlic powder and onion powder. Broil until the cheese is melted.

To Serve: Garnish with Italian seasoning and pepper.

Servings: 2

Cheese Course

To Serve: Arrange the pear wedges on a plate and spoon the ricotta over the pears. Garnish with cracked black pepper.

Servings: 2

2 pears, cored and cut into wedges

1 cup nonfat ricotta cheese

Cracked black pepper

Chicken and Swiss Bites

I ounce deli-style fat-free chicken breast, thinly sliced

4 ounces nonfat Swiss cheese, cut into strips

4 multigrain crackers

I cup salsa

To Serve: Roll the chicken slices around the Swiss cheese and arrange on top of the crackers. Garnish with salsa.

Servings: 2

Chicken Salad with Apples

1. In a small saucepan, cook the chicken in water until the chicken is fully cooked. Drain, cool, and dice the chicken.

2. In a mixing bowl, combine the chicken, apple, celery, sour cream, onion salt, and celery seeds. Cover and chill.

To Serve: Spoon the chicken salad into small bowls.

Servings: 2

2¾ ounces skinless, boneless chicken breast

2 cups peeled, cored, and diced Granny Smith apple

1¾ cups finely diced celery

1 cup nonfat sour cream

½ teaspoon celery seeds

1 tablespoon onion salt

Crunchy Celery Sticks with Roasted-Garlic Hummus and Smoked Turkey

I garlic clove, peeled

I cup cooked garbanzo beans, drained and rinsed

3 tablespoons freshly squeezed lemon juice

I stalk celery, cut into thick sticks

3 ounces deli-style sliced fat-free turkey

½ teaspoon olive oil

Salt and cracked black pepper to taste

I teaspoon dried parsley

1. Preheat the oven or toaster oven to 350°F. Wrap the garlic clove in foil and roast for 10 minutes. For the hummus, in a food processor, combine the roasted garlic, garbanzo beans, lemon juice, and olive oil. Pulse until a smooth paste forms. Season with salt and pepper. (If the hummus is too thick, add a little water until it reaches the desired consistency.)

To Serve: Arrange the celery sticks and turkey slices on plates. Serve the hummus in a small bowl and garnish with dried parsley.

Servings: 2

Edamame and Tuna Sashimi with Ginger-Scallion Vinaigrette

1. Cook edamame in boiling water for 2 minutes. Drain edamame and set aside. For vinaigrette, whisk together the water, soy sauce, ginger, and scallion. Toss the shredded carrots and tuna slices with the vinaigrette.

To Serve: Place the warm edamame in the center of a plate and season with a little salt. Arrange the carrots and tuna slices around the edamame.

Servings: 2

NOTE: Combining warm edamame with chilled tuna makes a refreshing hot and cold snack.

⅓ cup edamame beans, removed from pods

3 teaspoons grated ginger

3 teaspoons slivered scallion

3 cups shredded carrots

2¼ ounces sushi-grade yellowfin tuna, thinly sliced

½ cup water

1 tablespoon soy sauce

Salt to taste

Grilled Chicken Kabobs with Carrot-Ginger Vinaigrette

1¾ cups shredded carrots

I Granny Smith apple, shredded

½ cup rice wine vinegar

5 ounces skinless, boneless chicken breast, cut into bite-size pieces

I bell pepper, seeded and cut into squares

I teaspoon ground ginger

Salt and cracked black pepper to taste

Cooking oil spray

1. In a blender or food processor, combine the carrots, apple, rice wine vinegar, ginger, salt, and cracked black pepper. Pulse until smooth. Pour into a container and refrigerate. If the vinaigrette is too thick, add a little water.

2. Alternately thread chicken and bell pepper pieces onto skewers. Coat lightly with cooking spray and season with salt and cracked black pepper. On a hot nonstick grill pan, cook the chicken skewers for 10 minutes or until the chicken is fully cooked.

To Serve: Place the chicken kabobs on plates and drizzle with the vinaigrette. Serve warm.

Servings: 2

NOTE: If you double this snack, you'll have a great lunch.

Chicken Slices with Cheese and Crackers

To Serve: Arrange the crackers on a plate and serve with chicken, cheese, and fruit slices.

Servings: 2

6 whole grain crackers or any high-fiber, low-sugar crackers

2 ounces deli-style smoked chicken, thinly sliced

2 ounces nonfat cheddar cheese, thinly sliced

½ peach, cored and thinly sliced

½ pear, pitted and thinly sliced

Pear and Arugula Salad with Ricotta

I strip turkey bacon

1½ cups arugula leaves

2 pears, cored and thinly sliced

¾ cup nonfat ricotta cheese, softened

I lemon, cut in half

Salt and cracked black pepper to taste

1. Microwave the turkey bacon for 2 minutes or until crisp. Crumble the bacon.

To Serve: Arrange the arugula on plates and top with the pear slices and crumbled turkey bacon. Spoon the ricotta around the plates. Squeeze the juice from the lemon over the salad. Season with salt and pepper.

Servings: 2

Roasted Asparagus Spears with Turkey Slices

1. Preheat the toaster oven to 350°F.

2. Toss the asparagus spears with cooking spray, salt, and pepper. Roast in the toaster oven for 4 minutes.

To Serve: Lay the turkey slices on a cutting board. Sprinkle with the shredded carrots and place roasted asparagus spears in the middle. Roll the turkey tightly around the carrots and asparagus. Garnish with sliced onion.

Servings: 2

20 asparagus spears

6 ounces deli-style fat-free turkey, thinly sliced

2 cups shredded carrots

½ cup very thinly sliced red onion

Cooking oil spray

Salt and cracked black pepper to taste

Smoked Turkey and Fruit Salad

1½ cups quartered strawberries

1 cup orange sections

1 Granny Smith apple, cut into wedges

1 ounce smoked turkey, cut into cubes

½ cup nonfat cottage cheese

1. Gently toss together the strawberries, orange sections, apple wedges, and turkey cubes. Refrigerate until ready to serve.

To Serve: Spoon the cottage cheese into bowls and top with the fruit mixture.

Servings: 2

Salmon Sashimi with Plums

1. Whisk together the soy sauce, garlic, ginger, wasabi powder, and sugar substitute.

2. Arrange half of the plums on a plate. Arrange all of the salmon over the plums. Arrange the remaining plums over the salmon. Pour the soy mixture over the plums. Refrigerate.

To Serve: Garnish with scallion and sesame seeds.

Servings: 2

I clove garlic, mashed

12 ounces plums, pitted and thinly sliced

3 ounces fresh salmon, sliced paper-thin

I scallion, thinly sliced

¼ cup low-sodium soy sauce

I teaspoon ground ginger

½ teaspoon wasabi powder

½ teaspoon sugar substitute

2 teaspoons sesame seeds

Egg Salad with Toast Points

4 hard-boiled eggs, yolks removed

I hard-boiled egg

2 tablespoons nonfat mayonnaise

2 stalks celery, finely diced

2 slices whole grain bread, toasted

I teaspoon onion powder

I pinch celery seeds

Salt and cracked black pepper to taste

1. Chop the egg whites and whole egg and place in a mixing bowl. Stir in the mayonnaise, celery, onion powder, celery seeds, salt, and pepper. Mix well.

To Serve: Cut the toast into quarters and serve with egg salad.

Servings: 2

Egg and Celery Platter with Mustard-Balsamic Sauce

1. Quarter the egg whites and set aside. Whisk together the sour cream, balsamic vinegar, mustard, salt, and pepper.

To Serve: Arrange the egg whites and celery sticks on a plate. Drizzle with the sauce and garnish with pepper.

Servings: 2

3 hard-boiled eggs, yolks removed

1¾ cups nonfat sour cream

½ cup balsamic vinegar

3 teaspoons Dijon mustard

4 stalks celery, cut into small sticks

Salt and cracked black pepper to taste

Hard-Boiled Eggs Stuffed with Tuna Salad

½ cup canned water-pack tuna, drained

½ cup nonfat sour cream

¼ cup thinly sliced scallions

2 hard-boiled eggs, halved and yolks removed

3 cups shredded carrots

I teaspoon onion powder

I teaspoon garlic powder

Salt and cracked black pepper to taste

1. In a bowl, combine the tuna, sour cream, scallions, onion powder, garlic powder, salt, and pepper. Stir until the ingredients are combined. Stuff the egg whites with the tuna mixture.

To Serve: Make a shredded carrot nest on a plate and top with the stuffed eggs. Garnish with pepper.

Servings: 2

Spinach Frittata and Toast

1. Whisk together the egg whites, onion powder, garlic salt, and pepper. Coat a nonstick skillet with cooking spray and heat the skillet. Add the egg white mixture and cook until it begins to set. Add the spinach and cover the pan. Cook until the eggs begin to set on top. Sprinkle the cheese over the frittata and cook until cheese is melted.

To Serve: Cut frittata into wedges and serve hot or cold with toast.

Servings: 2

½ cup egg whites

4 cups spinach

2 tablespoons shredded part-skim-milk mozzarella cheese

4 slices whole wheat bread, toasted

1 pinch onion powder

1 pinch garlic salt

Cracked black pepper to taste

Olive oil cooking spray

Hot Dog Skewers with Cherry Tomatoes and Pickles

4 veggie hot dogs

3 cups halved button mushrooms

2 cups cherry tomatoes

I cup pickles cut into chunks

3 tablespoons Dijon mustard

1. Microwave the veggie hot dogs for 1½ minutes. Cut each hot dog into four pieces. Alternately thread hot dog pieces, mushrooms, tomatoes, and pickles on skewers.

To Serve: Serve warm or cold with Dijon mustard.

Servings: 2

Roast Beef with Carrot-Pear Slaw

1. Lightly toss together the shredded carrots, pear, and lime juice. Combine the sour cream and horseradish and gently stir into the carrot mixture.

To Serve: Season the roast beef with salt and pepper and serve with the coleslaw.

Servings: 2

1½ cups shredded carrots

1 pear, cored and chopped

¼ cup nonfat sour cream

1 tablespoon horseradish

4 ounces deli-style roast beef, thinly sliced

1 teaspoon lime juice

Salt and cracked black pepper to taste

Spicy Jumbo Shrimp with Black Bean Dip

6 jumbo shrimp, peeled and deveined

1⅓ cups canned black beans, drained

¼ cup finely diced red onion

1 lime

4 tablespoons whole cilantro leaves

1 teaspoon red pepper flakes

Salt and cracked black pepper to taste

Cooking oil spray

1. Season the shrimp with half of the red pepper flakes, salt, and cracked black pepper. Coat a nonstick skillet with cooking spray and heat skillet. Add the shrimp and cook for 2 minutes or until the shrimp turn opaque.

2. Combine the black beans and red onion with the juice from one half of the lime, cilantro, remaining red pepper flakes, salt, and cracked black pepper.

To Serve: Place the black bean mixture in a bowl and serve with the shrimp. Slice the remaining lime half and garnish with the lime slices.

Servings: 2

Carrot Sticks with Onion Dip

1. Beat together the sour cream, cream cheese, and onion soup mix until very smooth.

To Serve: Arrange the carrot sticks on a plate and serve with the onion dip.

Servings: 2

¾ cup nonfat sour cream

½ cup nonfat cream cheese

1 tablespoon dry onion soup mix

12 ounces carrots, cut into sticks

Spinach Dip with Carrot Sticks

1¼ pounds spinach leaves

1 cup nonfat sour cream

¼ cup shredded nonfat mozzarella cheese

3 carrots, cut into 2-inch sticks

1 teaspoon onion powder

1 teaspoon garlic powder

Salt and cracked black pepper to taste

1. Combine the spinach, sour cream, mozzarella, onion powder, garlic powder, salt, and pepper in a plastic container. Microwave for 1½ minutes and stir.

To Serve: Serve the spinach dip with the carrot sticks.

Servings: 2

Smoked Salmon Mousse with Crackers

1. In a food processor, combine the smoked salmon, cream cheese, lemon juice, salt, and pepper. Pulse until smooth.

To Serve: Spoon the salmon mixture onto a plate and arrange the crackers around the plate. Garnish with dried dill and additional pepper.

Servings: 2

2 ounces smoked salmon

¼ cup nonfat cream cheese

6 tablespoons freshly squeezed lemon juice

6 multigrain crackers or any high-fiber, low-sugar crackers

Salt and cracked black pepper to taste

I teaspoon dried dill

White Bean Dip

½ cup nonfat cream cheese

⅓ cup drained white navy beans

1 tablespoon freshly squeezed lemon juice

1 stalk celery, cut into sticks

Salt and cracked black pepper to taste

1. In a food processor, combine cream cheese, navy beans, lemon juice, salt, and pepper. Pulse until a smooth paste forms.

To Serve: Arrange the celery sticks on a plate and serve with bean dip.

Servings: 2

Chips and Salsa

1. Preheat oven to 375°F. Put the tortilla triangles on a baking pan and bake until they are crisp. Set aside and cool.

To Serve: Place the tortillas in two shallow bowls. Dollop sour cream on the chips. Spoon the salsa over the sour cream. Sprinkle the cheddar cheese on top and garnish with scallion.

Servings: 2

3 large whole grain or whole wheat tortillas, cut into triangles

½ tablespoon nonfat sour cream

1 cup salsa

½ cup shredded nonfat cheddar cheese

1 scallion, thinly sliced

Pesto Crisps with Tomatoes and Cheese

¾ cup nonfat ricotta cheese

6 multigrain crackers (pesto or any Italian flavor)

8 small tomatoes, sliced

2 tablespoons basil leaves

Salt and cracked black pepper to taste

1. Spread a generous amount of ricotta on each cracker. Season the tomatoes with salt and arrange them on top of the crackers.

To Serve: Sprinkle the tomatoes with pepper and garnish with basil leaves.

Servings: 2

Sauteed Apples over Rice Cakes

1. Spray a nonstick skillet with cooking spray and heat the skillet. Add the apple wedges and cook until they begin to soften. Season apples with cinnamon.

To Serve: Place the rice cakes on plates and top with the cottage cheese. Arrange the apples over the cheese. Garnish with chopped turkey jerky.

Servings: 2

NOTE: The saltiness of the turkey jerky balances with the sweetness of the apples.

2 Granny Smith apples, peeled, cored, and cut into wedges

4 rice cakes

I tablespoon low-fat cottage cheese

1½ ounces smoked turkey jerky, finely chopped

Cooking oil spray

I pinch ground cinnamon

Pears with Peanut Butter Dip

⅓ cup nonfat cream cheese

2 teaspoons peanut butter

2 pears, cored and cut into wedges

1. Combine the cream cheese and peanut butter.

To Serve: Spoon the cream cheese mixture over the pear wedges.

Servings: 2

Cottage Cheese and Pears

1. Toss the pear wedges with the lemon juice. Combine the cottage cheese and the sugar substitute.

To Serve: Serve the pear wedges with the cottage cheese as a dip.

Servings: 2

2 pears, cored and cut into wedges

I teaspoon freshly squeezed lemon juice

I¼ cups nonfat cottage cheese

I½ teaspoons sugar substitute

Fruit Skewers with Cottage Cheese

I pear, cored and cut into cubes

I teaspoon freshly squeezed lemon juice

20 strawberries, stems removed

I peach, pitted and cut into cubes

1⅛ cups nonfat cottage cheese

1. Lightly toss the pear cubes with the lemon juice.

2. Thread the pear cubes, strawberries, and peach cubes onto skewers. Chill until serving.

To Serve: Serve the fruit skewers with the cottage cheese.

Servings: 2

NOTE: You may also choose other 5-Factor-friendly fruits for this recipe.

Strawberry-Oatmeal Bars with Yogurt

1. Preheat the oven to 300°F. Combine the strawberries, rolled oats, egg whites, and 1 teaspoon of sugar substitute.

2. Coat a shallow baking dish with the cooking spray. Pour the strawberry mixture into the baking dish. Bake for 15 to 20 minutes. Set aside and cool.

3. Increase oven temperature to 425°F. Slice the cake into bars. Recoat the baking dish with cooking spray. Place the bars back in the baking dish. Bake for 5 minutes more or until crisp and golden. Cool.

To Serve: Stir the remaining sugar substitute into the yogurt. Serve the bars with yogurt for dipping.

Servings: 2

I cup sliced strawberries

½ cup rolled oats

½ cup egg whites

½ cup nonfat plain yogurt

2 teaspoons sugar substitute

Cooking oil spray

Toast with Berries and Cocoa Cottage Cheese

1 cup fresh berries

2 slices whole grain bread, toasted

½ cup low-fat cottage cheese

1 tablespoon unsweetened cocoa powder

2 teaspoons sugar substitute

1. Crush the berries with a fork and spoon them over the toast. Combine the cottage cheese, cocoa powder, and sugar substitute.

To Serve: Serve the toast with berries with the cottage cheese.

Servings: 2

Butterscotch and Apple Pudding

1. Place the apple in a container with 2 tablespoons water. Microwave for 2 minutes and set aside to cool. Whisk the pudding mix and the milk until smooth. Fold in the apple.

To Serve: Spoon ½ cup of ricotta cheese into each of two small glass bowls. Spoon the instant pudding on top.

Servings: 2

I Fuji apple, peeled, cored, and diced

I packet sugar-free, fat-free butterscotch instant pudding mix

1½ cups cold nonfat milk

I cup nonfat ricotta cheese, softened

Cheesecake

1½ tablespoons unflavored gelatin powder

½ cup nonfat cream cheese

½ cup nonfat sour cream

3 cups strawberries

¼ cup water

3 teaspoons sugar substitute

3 teaspoons vanilla extract

1. In a bowl, dissolve the gelatin powder in the water. Stir in the cream cheese, sour cream, sugar substitute, and vanilla extract. Pour the gelatin mixture into a glass baking dish and refrigerate until set.

To Serve: Spoon cheesecake onto plates and top with strawberries.

Servings: 2

Chocolate-Berry Parfaits

1. Whisk together the chocolate pudding mix and nonfat milk until smooth. In another bowl, whisk together the cottage cheese, yogurt, and sugar substitute.

To Serve: Spoon 1 tablespoon of pudding into each serving glass. Top with 1 tablespoon of the cottage cheese mixture and several raspberries. Repeat until all ingredients are used. Garnish with additional raspberries.

Servings: 2

I package fat-free, sugar-free chocolate-flavor pudding mix

I cup nonfat milk

¾ cup nonfat cottage cheese

½ cup nonfat plain yogurt

1¼ cups fresh raspberries

I teaspoon sugar substitute

Espresso Panna Cotta

I cup nonfat plain yogurt

I cup nonfat sour cream or quark

I shot espresso coffee, chilled

I tablespoon finely chopped bittersweet chocolate

3 teaspoons vanilla extract

2 teaspoons sugar substitute

1. Whisk together the yogurt, sour cream, coffee, chopped chocolate, vanilla extract, and sugar substitute until smooth. Pour into two small containers and chill until ready to serve.

To Serve: Serve chilled.

Servings: 2

NOTE: If you want to avoid caffeine, use decaf espresso. You can also try adding a fat-free, sugar-free coffee flavoring such as hazelnut or Irish cream.

Fresh Figs with Balsamic Cream Sauce

1. In a food processor, combine the cottage cheese, sour cream, balsamic vinegar, and sugar substitute. Process until smooth.

To Serve: Arrange the fig quarters on plates and pour the sauce over the figs. Garnish with pepper.

Servings: 2

1 cup nonfat cottage cheese

2 tablespoons nonfat sour cream

½ tablespoon balsamic vinegar

6 figs, quartered

1 teaspoon sugar substitute

Cracked black pepper to taste

Apple Wedges with Cinnamon Cream

1 Granny Smith apple, cored and cut into wedges

1 teaspoon freshly squeezed lemon juice

1 cup nonfat sour cream

¾ cup nonfat cream cheese, softened

2 teaspoons ground cinnamon

2 teaspoons sugar substitute

1. Toss the apple wedges with the lemon juice. Whisk together the sour cream, cream cheese, cinnamon, and sugar substitute. Microwave for 30 seconds.

To Serve: Place the apple wedges on plates and top with the cinnamon cream.

Servings: 2

Sauteed Peaches with Cheese

1. Coat a nonstick skillet with cooking spray and heat the skillet. Place the peach wedges flat on the skillet and cook until they begin to soften. Turn each wedge over and cook other side.

To Serve: Spoon nonfat ricotta into small bowls and top with the peach wedges. Sprinkle with the sugar substitute and serve immediately.

Servings: 2

Note: If you do not have peaches, substitute apples or pears.

1⅜ pounds peaches, pitted and cut into wedges

1 cup nonfat ricotta cheese

Cooking oil spray

2 teaspoons sugar substitute

Gelatin with Berries and Yogurt

I package sugar-free raspberry-flavor gelatin

⅔ cup nonfat plain yogurt

3 cups quartered strawberries

2 cups raspberries

⅓ cup blueberries

1. Prepare the gelatin according to the package instructions. Pour the gelatin mixture into ice cream bowls and refrigerate until set.

To serve: Spoon yogurt on top of the gelatin and serve with strawberries, raspberries, and blueberries.

Servings: 2

Raspberry Gelatin with Cottage Cheese

1. Prepare the raspberry gelatin according to the package instructions. Pour the gelatin into pliable ice cube molds and place one raspberry in each cavity. Refrigerate until set.

To Serve: Unmold the gelatin cubes into a serving bowl. Gently toss the cottage cheese and remaining raspberries with the gelatin. Serve immediately.

Servings: 2

2 packages sugar-free raspberry-flavor gelatin

3½ cups fresh raspberries

1 cup nonfat cottage cheese

Lemon Yogurt with Kiwi

1 cup nonfat plain yogurt

1 cup nonfat sour cream

1 tablespoon freshly squeezed lemon juice

2 sprigs fresh mint

2 kiwifruits, peeled and diced

1 teaspoon sugar substitute

1. Whisk together the yogurt, sour cream, lemon juice, and sugar substitute. Chop one of the mint sprigs and combine with the kiwi.

To Serve: Place the yogurt mixture in small bowls and top with the kiwi. Garnish with the remaining mint leaves.

Servings: 2

Lemon Pie

1. In a bowl, dissolve the gelatin powder in the warm water. Stir in the cream cheese, sour cream, sugar substitute, and lemon extract until the mixture is smooth. Spoon into a pie plate and refrigerate until set.

To Serve: Spoon the lemon mixture into dishes and garnish with lemon zest.

Servings: 2

NOTE: Unflavored gelatin is sold in most markets in the pudding and gelatin section.

1 tablespoon unflavored gelatin powder

½ cup nonfat cream cheese, softened

½ cup nonfat sour cream

¼ cup warm water

2 teaspoons sugar substitute

2 teaspoons lemon extract

2 teaspoons lemon zest

Chocolate-Mint Shakes

3½ cups quartered strawberries

2¼ cups nonfat milk

¾ scoop protein powder

1 tablespoon unsweetened cocoa powder

1 sprig fresh mint

1½ teaspoons sugar substitute

Crushed ice

1. Place the strawberries, milk, protein powder, cocoa powder, sugar substitute, and mint in a blender and pulse until smooth.

To Serve: Pour over crushed ice in tall glasses and serve immediately.

Servings: 2

Passion Fruit and Tangerine Shakes

1. Cut the passion fruits in half and scoop out the pulp and seeds. Place the passion fruit, tangerine sections, protein powder, and sugar substitute in a blender. Add the milk and pulse until smooth.

To Serve: Pour over crushed ice in tall glasses.

Servings: 2

NOTE: If you are unable to find fresh passion fruits, buy passion fruit pulp from the frozen section of your local market.

8 passion fruits

I cup tangerine sections

2 scoops protein powder (100% whey)

2¾ cups nonfat milk

2 teaspoons sugar substitute

Crushed ice

Tropical Berry Protein Shakes

2 passion fruits

I cup raspberries

¾ cup nonfat milk

I scoop protein powder (100% whey)

3 teaspoons sugar substitute

½ cup water

Crushed ice

1. Cut the passion fruits in half and spoon out the pulp. In a blender, combine the passion fruit pulp, raspberries, milk, protein powder, and sugar substitute. Add the water and pulse until smooth.

To Serve: Pour over crushed ice in tall glasses.

Servings: 2

NOTE: If you are not able to find passion fruits in your local market, use 3 tablespoons freshly squeezed orange juice.

Berry Protein Shakes

1. Combine the milk, raspberries, strawberries, protein powder, and vanilla extract in a blender. Blend until smooth.

To Serve: Pour over crushed ice in tall glasses and serve immediately.

Servings: 2

NOTE: Look for 100% whey protein powder in health food stores or in the fitness section of your local market. Or use soy protein powder.

2 cups nonfat milk

1½ cups raspberries

1 cup strawberries

½ scoop protein powder (100% whey)

1 teaspoon vanilla extract

Crushed ice

Meal 3. Lunch

Antipasto

4 cups canned artichoke hearts, drained

2 cups diced tomatoes

¾ cup cubed nonfat mozzarella cheese

2 ounces deli-style fat-free turkey, cubed

I cup fat-free balsamic vinaigrette

Cracked black pepper to taste

I teaspoon dried basil

1. In a bowl, toss together artichoke hearts, tomatoes, cheese, turkey cubes, balsamic vinaigrette, and pepper. Garnish with dried basil.

Servings: 2

Baked Chicken and Black Bean Quesadillas with Salsa

1. Combine the cumin, paprika, garlic powder, salt, and pepper. Season the chicken breast with the spice mixture. Coat a nonstick skillet with cooking spray and heat the skillet. Add the chicken and cook on medium heat until brown, turning once. Cover the pan and cook for 3 minutes more or until the chicken is fully cooked. Cool the chicken and slice into strips.

2. Preheat the toaster oven to 350°F. Place one tortilla on a cutting board. Arrange the sliced chicken on the tortilla and top with the black beans and mozzarella. Cover with the other tortilla and press down. Bake until the cheese is melted.

To Serve: Cut the quesadilla into quarters and serve with salsa.

Servings: 2

2 ounces skinless, boneless chicken breast

2 whole grain or whole wheat tortillas

I cup canned black beans, rinsed and drained

½ cup shredded nonfat mozzarella cheese

2 cups salsa

½ tablespoon ground cumin

½ tablespoon paprika

I teaspoon garlic powder

Salt and cracked black pepper to taste

Cooking oil spray

Baked Potato Skins with Sloppy Joe

2 large sweet potatoes

6 ounces ground chicken breast

½ cup tomato sauce

½ cup ketchup

2 cups diced tomatoes

2 tablespoons sloppy joe seasoning

I tablespoon garlic powder

I teaspoon onion powder

Salt and cracked black pepper to taste

2 teaspoons dried chives

1. Preheat the oven to 375°F. Wrap the sweet potatoes in foil and bake until tender. Remove potatoes from the oven and let cool for 10 minutes. Slice the sweet potatoes in half lengthwise and scoop out three-fourths of the pulp. The skins must remain intact. Place the potato skins in the oven and bake for another 8 minutes. Remove and set aside.

2. In a saucepan, combine the ground chicken, tomato sauce, ketchup, sloppy joe seasoning, garlic powder, onion powder, salt, and pepper. Cook over medium heat for 15 minutes. Add the tomatoes; cook 5 minutes more.

To Serve: Place the potato skins on plates and ladle the sloppy joe mixture over the potato skins. Garnish with dried chives.

Servings: 2

Black Bean Gumbo

1. In a medium saucepan, combine the water, chicken broth, and cubed chicken breast. Simmer for 15 minutes. Add the black beans, tomatoes, and Cajun seasoning and cook for 3 minutes.

To Serve: Ladle the soup into bowls.

Servings: 2

NOTE: If the soup seems too thick, add a little more chicken broth or water.

I cup fat-free chicken broth

2 ounces skinless, boneless chicken breast, cut into cubes

3 cups canned black beans, drained

2 cups diced tomatoes

3 cups water

2 tablespoons Cajun seasoning

Chicken and Rice Miso Soup

4 cups fat-free chicken broth

2 ounces skinless, boneless chicken breast

2 tablespoons miso paste or instant miso soup

1¾ cups cooked brown rice

1 cup thinly sliced scallions

1. Combine the chicken broth, chicken breast, and miso paste or miso soup packet. Simmer about 20 minutes or until the chicken breast is no longer pink. Remove the chicken breast from the broth and dice it into small pieces.

2. Add the brown rice and the diced chicken to the soup and cook for 2 minutes.

To Serve: Ladle the soup into bowls and garnish with scallions.

Servings: 2

NOTE: Brown rice can be purchased precooked and heated 1 minute in the microwave. This alternative will save you time.

Chicken Fingers and French Fries

1. Preheat the oven or toaster oven to 375°F. Spread the sweet potato sticks on a sheet pan and lightly coat with cooking spray. Season with cinnamon, salt, and pepper. Bake for 25 minutes.

2. Dip the chicken strips into the egg whites, then drain off excess egg and coat with the ground bread. Coat a nonstick skillet with cooking spray and heat the skillet. Add the breaded chicken and cook until brown, turning once. Cook over medium-low heat for 5 minutes more.

3. Place the broccoli in a bowl with a little water and salt. Microwave for 2 minutes. Remove from the microwave and season with Mrs. Dash.

To Serve: Place the chicken fingers, sweet potato fries, and broccoli on plates.

Servings: 2

I large sweet potato, peeled and cut into sticks

5½ ounces skinless, boneless chicken breast, cut into strips

3 egg whites

4 slices stale whole grain bread, ground

4 cups broccoli florets

Cooking oil spray

I teaspoon ground cinnamon

Salt and cracked black pepper to taste

2 tablespoons Mrs. Dash Original Blend seasoning

Chinese Chicken Wraps with Peanut-Soy Sauce

5 ounces skinless, boneless chicken breast

I teaspoon unsalted peanut butter

¾ cup shredded carrots

4 large whole grain or whole wheat tortillas

¾ cup low-sodium soy sauce

I teaspoon ground ginger

I teaspoon ground coriander

I teaspoon dried chives

I teaspoon sugar substitute

1. Place the chicken breast in a saucepan, cover with water, and simmer until fully cooked. Remove from the heat and cut the chicken into small cubes.

2. Whisk together the soy sauce, ginger, coriander, chives, sugar substitute, and peanut butter. Place the chicken and shredded carrots in a Ziploc bag and add the soy sauce mixture. Seal and refrigerate for 15 minutes. Drain the chicken mixture.

To Serve: Place some of the chicken mixture on each tortilla. Roll tightly and cut into pieces. Serve warm or cold.

Servings: 2

Harley's Sweet Potato Melt

1. Microwave the sweet potatoes for 3½ minutes each or until tender. Cut in half and set aside.

2. Preheat the broiler or toaster oven broiler to medium. In a mixing bowl, combine the tuna, mayonnaise, Mrs. Dash, and lemon pepper.

To Serve: Place the tuna mixture on top of the sweet potato halves. Top with cheese and broil until the cheese has melted.

Servings: 2

Note: Tuna also comes with different flavorings. Try smoked tuna or tuna teriyaki by Starkist Creations.

2 large sweet potatoes

¾ cup water-pack canned tuna, drained

½ cup nonfat mayonnaise

½ cup shredded part-skim-milk mozzarella cheese

1 teaspoon Mrs. Dash roasted garlic and onion seasoning

Lemon pepper to taste

Mediterranean-Style Chicken and Quinoa Salad

6 ounces skinless, boneless chicken breast

¾ cup quinoa

1⅓ cups diced, seeded plum tomatoes

1 cup chopped fresh parsley

3 tablespoons freshly squeezed lemon juice

Salt and cracked black pepper to taste

1. Place the chicken breast and 2 cups of water in a small saucepan and cook for 8 minutes. Let the chicken cool and dice it. Set aside.

2. Put the quinoa and 1½ cups of water into a saucepan and simmer about 15 minutes or until the liquid is absorbed. Stir occasionally. Combine the chicken, quinoa, tomatoes, parsley, lemon juice, salt, and pepper; toss gently.

To Serve: Spoon the salad into shallow bowls.

Servings: 2

Mexican Chicken Salad with Spicy Salsa Dressing

1. Combine the fajita seasoning mix, cumin, salt, and pepper. Coat the chicken breast with the seasoning mixture. Microwave the chicken for 6 minutes. Remove from the microwave and set aside to cool slightly.

2. In a blender, combine the sour cream and salsa. Pulse until smooth. If the dressing is too thick, add a little water.

To Serve: Cut the chicken breast into ½-inch pieces and toss it with the lettuce, corn, and salsa dressing. Serve immediately.

Servings: 2

6 ounces skinless, boneless chicken breast

I cup nonfat sour cream

I cup salsa

I small head iceberg lettuce, coarsely chopped

1½ cups canned corn, drained

I teaspoon fajita seasoning mix

I pinch cumin

Salt and cracked black pepper to taste

Minestrone

4 cups chicken broth

2 cups canned stewed tomatoes

1⅓ cups thinly sliced button mushrooms

1⅓ cups cooked cannellini beans

1 cup diced smoked turkey breast

2 tablespoons dried basil

1 teaspoon sugar substitute

Salt and cracked black pepper to taste

1. In a saucepan combine the chicken broth, stewed tomatoes, sliced mushrooms, cannellini beans, turkey breast, basil, sugar substitute, salt, and pepper. Bring to a boil. Lower the temperature and simmer about 15 minutes or until the soup is reduced to half its volume.

To Serve: Ladle into soup bowls and serve immediately.

Servings: 2

Mixed Greens with Turkey and Cheese Quesadillas

1. Place the turkey slices on one side of each tortilla. Sprinkle with cheese and fold tortilla in half. Press tightly to secure the filling.

2. Coat a nonstick skillet with cooking spray and heat the skillet. Cook the tortillas for 1 minute on each side or until the cheese is melted. Slide the quesadillas onto a cutting board. Slice each into three or four triangles. Set aside.

To Serve: Toss the mixed greens with the salad dressing. Place the greens in the center of the plates. Arrange the quesadilla triangles around the salads.

Servings: 2

¼ pound deli-style sliced fat-free turkey

2 whole grain or whole wheat tortillas

½ cup shredded nonfat mozzarella cheese

3 cups mixed greens

I cup fat-free blue cheese salad dressing or other fat-free dressing

Cooking oil spray

Mushroom-Barley Risotto

3 cups sliced button mushrooms

I cup nonfat beef broth

½ cup pearl barley

3 ounces shrimp, peeled, deveined, and cut in half

I cup nonfat sour cream

4 cups water

I tablespoon dried sage

I tablespoon garlic powder

Salt and cracked black pepper to taste

1. In a large saucepan, combine the water, mushrooms, beef broth, and barley. Simmer for 15 minutes or until most of the liquid has been absorbed. Stir in the shrimp, sour cream, sage, garlic powder, salt, and pepper. Simmer for 2 minutes.

To Serve: Ladle the risotto into bowls and serve hot.

Servings: 2

Open-Face Turkey BLT

1. Microwave the turkey bacon for 3 minutes or until crisp. Crumble the bacon and set aside. Lay the romaine leaves flat on a plate. Layer with the sliced turkey, sliced tomatoes, and the turkey bacon. Season with salt and pepper and drizzle with red wine vinegar.

To Serve: Place the bun-less BLTs on plates and serve immediately.

Servings: 2

2 strips turkey bacon

I head romaine lettuce, leaves washed and patted dry

6 ounces deli-style fat-free turkey, thinly sliced

2 tomatoes, thinly sliced

I tablespoon red wine vinegar

Salt and cracked black pepper to taste

Pink Pizza

4 large whole grain or whole wheat tortillas

I cup tomato sauce

¾ cup nonfat ricotta cheese

I cup chopped sun-dried tomatoes

¾ cup shredded nonfat mozzarella cheese

1. Preheat the oven to 375°F. Place the tortillas on a baking sheet and bake for 2 minutes. Remove from the oven. Ladle half of the tomato sauce over the tortillas and spread with the ricotta cheese. Ladle on the remaining tomato sauce and sprinkle with sun-dried tomatoes and shredded mozzarella. Bake until the cheese is melted.

To Serve: Cut the pizzas into slices and serve immediately.

Servings: 2

Portobello and Turkey Stacks

1. Preheat the broiler to medium. Season the turkey breast with salt and pepper. Coat a nonstick skillet with cooking spray and heat the skillet. Add the turkey breast and cook until fully cooked, turning once. Slice thinly and set aside.

2. Lightly coat the mushroom caps with cooking spray and sprinkle with salt and pepper. Coat a nonstick skillet with cooking spray and heat the skillet. Add the mushrooms and cook until tender, turning once. Set aside.

To Assemble: Place the mushrooms on a sheet pan and top with the turkey. Place the tomato on top of the turkey and season with salt and pepper. Top with mozzarella. Broil until the cheese is melted.

To Serve: With a spatula, carefully slide the turkey stacks onto serving plates. Sprinkle with dried basil. Serve with crackers.

Servings: 2

4 ounces skinless, boneless turkey breast

4 portobello mushrooms, stems removed

1 tomato, thinly sliced

1 ounce fat-free mozzarella cheese, thinly sliced

10 whole grain or multigrain crackers

Salt and cracked black pepper to taste

Olive oil cooking spray

1 teaspoon dried basil

Salad Niçoise

12 ounces sweet potato

6 cups green beans, cooked

1½ cups water-pack tuna, drained

2 hard-boiled egg whites, chopped

½ cup fat-free Italian salad dressing

Salt and cracked black pepper to taste

1. Microwave the sweet potato for 3 minutes. Peel the potato and slice into ½-inch rounds. Set aside.

To Serve: Place the sweet potato rounds on serving plates. Arrange the green beans beside the sweet potato. Sprinkle the tuna and chopped egg whites around the green beans and sweet potatoes. Season with salt and pepper and drizzle with the salad dressing. Served chilled.

Servings: 2

Salmon Tartare with Arugula

1. In a bowl, combine the diced salmon, capers, juice from 1 of the lemons, onion and garlic salt, garlic powder, salt, and pepper.

To Serve: Arrange the arugula on a plate and season with salt and pepper. Sprinkle the salmon mixture over the arugula. Cut remaining lemon into wedges and garnish with wedges. Serve with crackers.

Servings: 2

6 ounces salmon fillets, finely diced

¼ cup capers, rinsed and chopped

2 lemons

I pound arugula

12 multigrain crackers

I tablespoon onion and garlic salt

I tablespoon garlic powder

Salt and cracked black pepper to taste

Greek-Style Shrimp and Spinach Salad

½ cup freshly squeezed lemon juice

1½ ounces feta cheese, crumbled

5 ounces shrimp, peeled and deveined

1 pound spinach leaves

4 cups orange sections

2 teaspoons ground oregano

1 teaspoon ground coriander

Salt and cracked black pepper to taste

1½ tablespoons Mrs. Dash seasoning

Cooking oil spray

1. Whisk together the lemon juice, feta cheese, oregano, coriander, salt, and pepper. Set aside. Season the shrimp with Mrs. Dash, salt, and pepper. Coat a nonstick skillet with cooking spray and heat the skillet until very hot. Add the shrimp and cook about 2 minutes or until shrimp are opaque.

To serve: Toss the feta mixture with the spinach and arrange on plates. Top with the shrimp and garnish with the orange sections.

Servings: 2

Smoked Salmon Pizza

1. Preheat the oven to 375°F. Place the tortillas on a baking sheet and bake for 4 minutes or until crisp.

To Serve: Spread the cream cheese on the tortillas and top with the tomato slices. Arrange the smoked salmon over the tomato and sprinkle with the red onion. Season with salt and pepper. Cut into wedges.

Servings: 2

4 whole grain or whole wheat tortillas

I cup nonfat cream cheese, softened

2 tomatoes, thinly sliced

4 ounces thinly sliced smoked salmon

⅔ cup thinly sliced red onion

Salt and cracked black pepper to taste

Snapper Ceviche with Sweet Potato Rounds

2 medium sweet potatoes

10 ounces thinly sliced snapper fillet

1¼ cups freshly squeezed lemon juice

½ cup thinly sliced red onion

3 tablespoons chopped fresh cilantro

1 teaspoon ground cumin

1 pinch sugar substitute

Salt and cracked black pepper to taste

1. Microwave the sweet potatoes for 3 minutes each. Let the sweet potatoes cool, then peel. Slice into ½-inch rounds and set aside.

2. In a Ziploc bag, combine the snapper, lemon juice, red onion, cilantro, cumin, sugar substitute, salt, and pepper. Marinate the fish in the refrigerator for 15 to 20 minutes or until it is completely pickled. (The fish will be white and firm to the bite.)

To Serve: Arrange the sweet potato rounds on plates and spoon the snapper mixture on top.

Servings: 2

Green Bean Salad with Tuna and Grapefruit-Scallion Vinaigrette

1. In a saucepan, cook the green beans with a pinch of salt in boiling water for 2 minutes. Drain the beans and place them in an ice bath until cool. Drain again.

2. In a bowl, whisk together the rice vinegar, ginger, garlic powder, sesame seeds, salt, and pepper. Add two grapefruit sections to the vinaigrette and whisk until the segments fall apart. Place the green beans in a large bowl and toss with the tuna, scallions, and vinaigrette.

To Serve: Place salad on plates and garnish with the remaining grapefruit segments.

Servings: 2

2 pounds green beans, stems removed

I cup rice wine vinegar

2 small grapefruit, sectioned

8 ounces canned tuna, drained and flaked

½ bunch scallions, bias sliced

I teaspoon ground ginger

I teaspoon garlic powder

I teaspoon sesame seeds

Salt and cracked black pepper to taste

Stuffed Mushrooms and Greens

2 cups lump crabmeat

1¾ cups prepared bulgur

6 large button mushroom caps

5 cups mixed greens

½ cup fat-free red wine vinaigrette salad dressing

2 teaspoons paprika

I teaspoon dried mint

I teaspoon garlic powder

I teaspoon onion salt

Salt and cracked black pepper to taste

Cooking oil spray

1. Preheat the oven to 375°F. Combine crabmeat, bulgur, paprika, mint, garlic powder, onion salt, salt, and pepper. It should be just moist enough to hold together. Pack the crab and bulgur mixture into each mushroom cap. Lightly coat with cooking spray. Place in a baking pan and bake for 10 minutes.

To Serve: Season the greens with salt and pepper and toss with the red wine vinaigrette. Arrange the greens on plates and put the warm mushrooms on top. Serve immediately.

Servings: 2

NOTE: To prepare the bulgur, soak it in 3 cups water for 20 minutes, then drain.

Tuscan Tomato Soup

1. Preheat the oven to 400°F. Place tomatoes in a baking dish and lightly coat with cooking spray. Roast for 15 minutes. Remove from the oven and set aside.

2. In a saucepan, combine the chicken broth, garlic powder, onion powder, sugar substitute, salt, and pepper. Simmer the mixture until it is reduced to half its volume. In a blender, pulse the tomatoes until chunky. Stir the tomatoes into the chicken broth mixture. Whisk in the sour cream.

To Serve: Ladle the soup into bowls and garnish with dried basil.

Servings: 2

1 cup canned stewed tomatoes

4 cups chicken broth

3 cups nonfat sour cream

Cooking oil spray

1 tablespoon garlic powder

1 tablespoon onion powder

1 teaspoon sugar substitute

Salt and cracked black pepper to taste

1 tablespoon dried basil

Meal 5. Dinner

5-Factor Lasagna

2 small eggplants, thinly sliced lengthwise

I cup tomato sauce

I pound tomatoes, thinly sliced

I cup nonfat ricotta cheese, softened

¾ cup shredded nonfat mozzarella cheese

Salt and cracked black pepper to taste

Cooking oil spray

2 tablespoons dried basil

2 tablespoons Italian seasoning

1. Preheat the oven to 400°F. Season the eggplant slices with salt and pepper and roast for 15 minutes.

2. Coat a glass baking dish with cooking spray and cover the bottom with eggplant slices. Ladle some of the tomato sauce over the eggplant and top with some of the tomato slices. Sprinkle the tomato slices with basil, Italian seasoning, salt, and pepper. Spread ricotta over the tomatoes. Sprinkle with shredded mozzarella. Repeat the layers, ending with mozzarella.

3. Bake for 20 minutes. Increase the heat to broil until the cheese turns golden.

To Serve: Cut the lasagna into slices and garnish with additional Italian seasoning.

Servings: 2

Argentine-Style Steak Salad with Watercress and Mustard-Cilantro Vinaigrette

1. In a mixing bowl, whisk together the vinegar, Dijon mustard, cilantro, salt, and pepper. Set aside.

2. Season the bison steak with cumin, coriander, salt, and pepper. Coat a nonstick skillet with cooking spray and heat the skillet. Add the steak and sear on each side to desired doneness, turning once. Remove the steak from the skillet and let stand for 1 minute. Slice the steak.

To Serve: Toss the watercress with the vinaigrette and place it on plates. Top with steak slices and garnish with radish slices.

Servings: 2

NOTE: Bison is a very lean meat, and has the best flavor and texture when cooked to medium-rare.

¼ cup white wine vinegar

1½ teaspoons Dijon mustard

6 ounces bison steak

4 bunches watercress, washed and patted dry

5 radishes, thinly sliced

2 tablespoons dried cilantro

Salt and cracked black pepper to taste

1 teaspoon ground cumin

1 teaspoon ground coriander

Cooking oil spray

Chicken Chow Mein

6 ounces skinless, boneless chicken breast, cut into strips

5 cups thinly sliced carrots

3 cups snow peas, stems removed

2 cups bean sprouts

Cooking oil spray

I tablespoon sesame seeds

I tablespoon garlic powder

½ cup low-sodium soy sauce

1. Coat a wok with cooking spray and heat the wok. Add the chicken strips and stir-fry for 2 minutes. Add the carrots, snow peas, bean sprouts, sesame seeds, and garlic powder. Stir-fry for 1 minute. Add the soy sauce and cook for 1 minute.

To Serve: Ladle into shallow bowls and garnish with a few additional sesame seeds.

Servings: 2

Chicken Ropa Vieja

1. In a saucepan, bring salted water to a boil. Add the chicken and cook over medium heat for 10 to 15 minutes. Drain the cooked chicken and cool. Shred the chicken.

2. In a saucepan, combine the tomato sauce, bell pepper slices, cumin, sugar substitute, bay leaf, salt, and cracked black pepper. Add the shredded chicken and cook for 5 minutes. Microwave the corn for 2 minutes. Season with salt and cracked black pepper. Discard bay leaf.

To Serve: Spoon the chicken mixture into bowls and top with corn. Garnish with fresh cilantro.

Servings: 2

7½ ounces skinless, boneless chicken breast

12 ounces tomato sauce

1 red bell pepper, seeded and thinly sliced

2½ cups canned corn, drained

2 tablespoons cilantro leaves

1 teaspoon ground cumin

1 teaspoon sugar substitute

1 bay leaf

Salt and cracked black pepper to taste

Chiles Rellenos with Brown Rice

2 large poblano peppers

6 ounces ground turkey breast

½ cup canned black beans, rinsed and drained

3 tablespoons tomato paste

1½ cups cooked brown rice

Cooking oil spray

I tablespoon ground cumin

I pinch sugar substitute

Salt and cracked black pepper to taste

1. Preheat the oven to 400°F. Lightly coat the poblanos with cooking spray. Place them on a baking sheet and roast for 20 minutes or until the skins begin to char. Remove the peppers from the heat. Immediately place them in a bowl and cover with plastic wrap to cool.

2. Carefully peel the poblanos and slit each one through one side. Remove the seeds with a paring knife and rinse the peppers under cold water to wash out any remaining seeds. Leave the peppers as intact as possible. Set the peppers aside.

3. Coat a nonstick skillet with cooking spray and heat skillet. Add the ground turkey and cook until no longer pink. Add the black beans, tomato paste, cumin, sugar substitute, salt, and cracked black pepper. Stir until well mixed. Spoon the turkey filling into the peppers.

To Serve: Spoon the cooked rice onto plates and top with the chiles. Garnish with fresh cilantro leaves, if desired.

Servings: 2

Country-Style Ham Steaks with Yams and Corn on the Cob

1. Coat a nonstick skillet with cooking spray and heat the skillet. Add the ham steaks and sear on each side until golden brown. Microwave the yams for about 3½ minutes each. Peel and slice them into rounds and season with salt and pepper. Cook the corn in boiling water for 3 minutes.

To Serve: Place the ham steaks on plates and serve with sliced yams and corn on the cob.

Servings: 2

9 ounces ham steaks

2 large yams

3 ears corn on the cob, husked and cut in half

Cooking oil spray

Salt and cracked black pepper to taste

Cream of Broccoli Soup with Sauteed Shrimp

2⅛ cups chicken broth

8 ounces broccoli florets

2¼ cups chopped carrots

¾ cup leeks, white part only, coarsely chopped

8 ounces shrimp, peeled, deveined, and cut into pieces

1 tablespoon garlic powder

Salt and cracked black pepper to taste

Cooking oil spray

1. In a large saucepan, bring the chicken broth to a boil and add the broccoli, carrots, leeks, garlic powder, salt, and pepper. Cook for 3 minutes or until the broccoli is bright green and tender to the fork. Remove from the heat and let cool slightly.

2. Ladle a portion of the broccoli mixture into a blender and pulse until it reaches a creamy consistency. Pour the blended soup into a large saucepan. Repeat until all the broccoli mixture is blended. Reheat the soup.

3. Coat a nonstick skillet with cooking spray and heat the skillet. Add the shrimp and season with salt and pepper. Cook about 2 minutes.

To Serve: Ladle the soup into bowls and garnish with shrimp.

Servings: 2

Creamy Lemon-Ginger Halibut with Corn on the Cob

1. Zest one lemon and squeeze out the juice. Whisk together the lemon zest, lemon juice, yogurt, coriander, ginger, salt, and pepper. Place the halibut fillets in a Ziploc bag and pour three-fourths of the yogurt mixture over the fish. Marinate for 5 minutes.

2. Meanwhile, place the corn in a plastic container with water. Microwave for 5 minutes. Season with salt and pepper and set aside.

3. Remove the fish from the marinade and place in a plastic container. Cover and microwave for 6 minutes or until fish flakes when tested with a fork.

To Serve: Place the fish and corn on plates. Spoon a little of the remaining yogurt mixture over the fish. Cut the remaining lemon into wedges and serve with fish.

Servings: 2

2 lemons

¾ cup nonfat plain yogurt

8 ounces boneless halibut fillet, cut into two portions

2 ears corn on the cob, husks removed

1 teaspoon ground coriander

1½ teaspoons ground ginger

Salt and cracked black pepper to taste

Crispy Chicken Tostadas

6 ounces skinless, boneless chicken breast

1½ cups thinly sliced Spanish onion

2 tablespoons freshly squeezed lime juice

4 medium whole grain or whole wheat tortillas

2 tablespoons nonfat sour cream

Salt and cracked black pepper to taste

1 teaspoon olive oil

4 teaspoons dried cilantro

1 teaspoon ground cumin

1. Place chicken in large saucepan and add water to cover, salt, and pepper. Cook over medium heat for 25 minutes or until the chicken is fully cooked. Remove the chicken, cool, and shred.

2. Heat the olive oil in a nonstick skillet. Add the onion and cook for 1 minute. Add the shredded chicken and stir constantly until it crisps. When most of the liquid has evaporated, drizzle the lime juice over the chicken and season with cilantro, cumin, salt, and pepper. Set aside. Bake the tortillas in a 350° oven until they are crisp and light golden.

To Serve: Place the tortillas on plates. Top with the chicken and sour cream.

Servings: 2

Bison Steak with Cauliflower-Carrot Mash and Brown Rice

1. In a medium saucepan, cook the carrots in lightly salted boiling water for 2 minutes. Add the cauliflower and cook for 3 minutes or until the cauliflower is tender. Drain the vegetables and place in a food processor. Pulse the vegetables with the sour cream, onion powder, salt, and pepper. Transfer to a bowl with lid and set aside.

2. Divide the steak into two portions. Season the steaks with steak seasoning, salt, and pepper. Coat a nonstick skillet with cooking spray and heat the skillet until very hot. Add the steaks and sear on both sides. Then reduce heat to medium-high and cook until they reach the desired doneness (bison is best served medium-rare). Remove from the heat and let the steaks stand for 1 minute.

To Serve: Place the cauliflower-carrot mash in the center of the plates. Slice the bison steaks and arrange the slices over the mash. Serve with brown rice.

Servings: 2

2¼ cups chopped carrots

3½ cups cauliflower florets

2 tablespoons nonfat sour cream

6½ ounces bison steak

1¼ cups cooked brown rice

1 tablespoon onion powder

Salt and cracked black pepper to taste

2 tablespoons Montreal steak seasoning

Cooking oil spray

Indian-Style Chicken with Curried Yogurt Sauce and Brown Rice

½ cup nonfat plain yogurt

1 teaspoon curry powder

8 ounces skinless, boneless chicken breast, butterflied and thinly pounded

2 cups cooked brown rice

2½ cups thinly sliced, peeled cucumber

½ teaspoon ground coriander

⅛ teaspoon ground paprika

Salt and cracked black pepper to taste

Cooking oil spray

1. Combine the yogurt, curry powder, coriander, paprika, salt, and pepper. Pour three-fourths of the mixture into a Ziploc bag. Add the chicken, seal, and refrigerate for 20 minutes. Drain the chicken and discard the marinade. Coat a nonstick skillet with cooking spray and heat the skillet. Add the chicken and sear on each side until golden brown. Cover the pan and reduce the heat to medium. Cook for 1 minute more and remove from the heat.

To Serve: Place the chicken and brown rice on plates. Top the chicken with the remaining yogurt sauce and the sliced cucumbers.

Servings: 2

Lobster and Peas with Tomato-Basil Sauce and Barley

1. In a soup pot, combine the tomato sauce, barley, lobster, basil, seafood seasoning mix, sugar substitute, salt, and pepper. Cook and stir for 4 minutes. Taste and adjust the seasonings. Add the peas and cook for 1 to 2 minutes.

To Serve: Ladle into shallow bowls and garnish with additional fresh basil leaves.

Servings: 2

NOTE: For a less expensive dish, you can prepare this recipe with shrimp or chicken breast.

1½ cups tomato sauce

1¼ cups cooked barley

1¼ cups uncooked lobster, coarsely chopped

½ bunch fresh basil, chopped

1½ cups frozen green peas

1 teaspoon seafood seasoning mix

1 teaspoon sugar substitute

Salt and cracked black pepper to taste

Salmon with Cucumber-Dill Salad

9 ounces salmon steak

2 large sweet potatoes

½ cup nonfat sour cream

2 tablespoons chopped fresh dill

I cup thinly sliced, peeled cucumber

½ tablespoon lemon pepper

I teaspoon paprika

Salt and cracked black pepper to taste

Cooking oil spray

1. Cut the salmon steak into two portions and season with lemon pepper, paprika, and salt. Coat a nonstick skillet with cooking spray and heat the skillet. Place the salmon steaks in the skillet, skin sides up. Sear for 1 minute, then turn and cook until the salmon flakes when tested with a fork.

2. Microwave the sweet potatoes for 3½ minutes each or until tender. Peel and slice into thick rounds. Season with salt and pepper and set aside.

3. Meanwhile, whisk together the sour cream, dill, salt, and pepper. Stir in the cucumber slices.

To Serve: Spoon the cucumber mixture over the salmon. Serve with sweet potato rounds.

Servings: 2

Scallop Ratatouille

1. In a soup pot, combine the tomatoes, zucchini, eggplant, mushrooms, water, basil, oregano, sugar substitute, salt, and pepper. Cover and cook over medium heat for 5 minutes. Add the scallops and cook for 2½ minutes more.

To Serve: Ladle the soup into bowls and garnish with additional dried basil.

Servings: 2

3 cups canned crushed tomatoes

3 cups cubed zucchini

3 cups cubed eggplant

3 cups quartered button mushrooms

½ pound small scallops

1 ½ cups water

3 tablespoons dried basil

2 tablespoons dried oregano

1 pinch sugar substitute

Salt and cracked black pepper to taste

Seared Halibut with Creamed Spinach and Brown Rice

5 ounces halibut fillets

I pound spinach leaves

½ cup nonfat cream cheese

¼ cup nonfat sour cream

1⅔ cups cooked brown rice

I teaspoon lemon pepper

Salt and cracked black pepper to taste

Cooking oil spray

I tablespoon onion powder

2 teaspoons garlic powder

1. Season the halibut fillets with lemon pepper and salt. Coat a nonstick skillet with cooking spray and heat the skillet. Add the halibut and sear on each side. Then cover the pan and cook until the fish flakes when tested with a fork. Set aside.

2. Cook the spinach in a nonstick pan over medium heat until wilted. Transfer the spinach to a strainer and press out as much liquid as possible.

3. Return the spinach to the pan. Add the cream cheese, sour cream, onion powder, garlic powder, salt, and cracked black pepper. Cook and stir over medium heat until hot.

4. Microwave the brown rice for 1 minute.

To Serve: Place the brown rice on the center of each plate. Top with halibut and spoon the creamed spinach over the halibut.

Servings: 2

Seared Scallops with Orange Sauce and Broccoli-Cauliflower Saute

1. Coat a nonstick skillet with cooking spray and heat the skillet. Add the scallops and season with the curry powder, salt, and pepper. Cook until scallops are golden brown. Add the broccoli, cauliflower, and orange juice. Cook until the broccoli is bright green and tender to the fork.

To serve: Spoon the scallops and vegetables into shallow bowls. Drizzle with the orange sauce.

Servings: 2

10 ounces large scallops

I pound broccoli florets

I pound cauliflower florets

I cup freshly squeezed orange juice

Cooking oil spray

I teaspoon curry powder

Salt and cracked black pepper to taste

Shrimp and Tofu Soup

1½ cups cooked brown rice

4 ounces shrimp, peeled, deveined, and cut in half

4 ounces firm tofu cut into 1-inch cubes

3 tablespoons miso paste or instant miso soup

4 cups water

1 cup low-sodium soy sauce

1. In a large saucepan, combine the water, rice, soy sauce, shrimp, tofu, and miso. Simmer for 2 minutes or until the shrimp are opaque.

To Serve: Ladle into soup bowls.

Servings: 2

Shrimp and Rice Stir-Fry

1. Remove the tails from the shrimp and cut the shrimp into bite-size pieces.

2. Coat a nonstick skillet with cooking spray and heat the skillet. Add the shrimp and cook for 2 minutes. Remove from the heat and set the shrimp aside.

3. Coat the skillet with cooking spray and heat the skillet. Add the rice and garlic powder and cook for 1 minute, stirring constantly. Add the broccoli and cook until it is bright green. Add the shrimp, scallions, soy sauce, and sesame seeds. Cook for 1 minute longer.

To Serve: Spoon the stir-fried mixture onto plates.

Servings: 2

I pound shrimp, peeled and deveined

1½ cups cooked brown rice

2 cups broccoli florets

¼ cup slivered scallions

Cooking oil spray

½ tablespoon garlic powder

¼ cup low-sodium soy sauce

2 teaspoons sesame seeds

Southern-Style Baked Chicken with Black-Eyed Peas and Collard Greens

6 ounces skinless, boneless chicken breast

5 bunches collard greens, cut into strips

2 cloves garlic, minced

¼ cup balsamic vinegar

2¾ cups canned black-eyed peas, drained and rinsed

1 tablespoon Lawry's Seasoned Salt

Cooking oil spray

¼ cup water

1 teaspoon sugar substitute

Salt and cracked black pepper to taste

1. Preheat the oven to 375°F.

2. Sprinkle the chicken with seasoned salt. Coat a nonstick skillet with cooking spray and heat the skillet. Sear the chicken on both sides until golden and crisp around the edges. Put the chicken in a baking dish and bake for 10 minutes.

3. Coat a large nonstick skillet with cooking spray and heat the skillet. Add the collard greens and garlic and cook for 4 minutes or until the greens are bright green. Add the vinegar and water. Cook until most of the liquid has evaporated. Add the sugar substitute, salt, and pepper and set the greens aside.

4. Place the black-eyed peas in a bowl and season with salt and pepper. Microwave for 1 minute.

To Serve: Transfer the hot chicken breasts to a cutting board and cut into ½-inch slices. Place the collard greens on the plates and arrange the chicken slices on top. Ladle the black-eyed peas over the chicken.

Servings: 2

Soy-Poached Chicken with Vegetables and Brown Rice

1. In a saucepan, combine the chicken, water, and soy sauce. Simmer for 8 minutes or until chicken is no longer pink. Drain the chicken and set aside.

2. Meanwhile, remove edamame beans from the pods and cook in boiling water for 2 minutes. Place the carrots, ginger, and garlic powder in a container and microwave for 2 minutes. Drain the edamame beans and stir into the carrot mixture. Season with a little salt.

To Serve: Place the chicken on plates and spoon the cooked brown rice on top. Garnish with the vegetable mixture.

Servings: 2

8 ounces skinless, boneless chicken breast, pounded thin

I cup edamame beans

2 cups thinly sliced carrots

1¼ cups cooked brown rice

2 cups water

I cup low-sodium soy sauce

I teaspoon ground ginger

I teaspoon garlic powder

Salt to taste

Spaghetti and Meatballs

2 small spaghetti squash, cut in half
and seeded

I cup canned crushed tomatoes

6 ounces ground turkey breast

I egg white

4 slices whole grain bread, toasted and
ground into crumbs

Cooking oil spray

Salt and cracked black pepper to taste

I bay leaf

I tablespoon sugar substitute

2 teaspoons onion powder

2 teaspoons garlic powder

I teaspoon tomato paste

Chopped fresh parsley (optional)

1. Preheat the oven to 400°F. Lightly coat the squash with cooking spray and season with salt and pepper. Bake for 30 minutes or until tender. (Or microwave each squash half for 6 minutes).

3. In a saucepan, combine the tomatoes, bay leaf, sugar substitute, 1 teaspoon of the onion powder, 1 teaspoon of the garlic powder, salt, and pepper. Bring to a simmer. In a mixing bowl, combine the ground turkey, egg white, bread crumbs, tomato paste, remaining onion powder, remaining garlic powder, salt, and pepper. Mix well. Roll 1½-inch meatballs between the palms of your hands. Drop the meatballs into the tomato sauce and cook for 15 minutes.

To Serve: Shred the spaghetti squash with forks and place on plates. Ladle meatballs and tomato sauce over the squash. Sprinkle with chopped parsley, if desired.

Servings: 2

Turkey Fajitas

1. Coat a nonstick skillet with cooking spray and heat the skillet. Add the turkey strips and cook for 2 minutes. Add the onion and cook 1 minute longer. Add the bell pepper, fajita seasoning mix, garlic powder, chili powder, salt, and cracked black pepper. Stir well to mix and cook for 1 minute.

To Serve: Heat the tortillas in the microwave for 15 seconds. Spoon the turkey mixture onto the tortillas and garnish with sour cream.

Servings: 2

6 ounces skinless, boneless turkey breast, cut into strips

I cup sliced Spanish onion

I bell pepper, seeded and cut into strips

2 large whole grain or whole wheat tortillas

½ cup nonfat sour cream

Cooking oil spray

2 tablespoons fajita seasoning mix

I tablespoon garlic powder

2 teaspoons chili powder

Salt and cracked black pepper to taste

Warm White Bean, Beet, and Turkey Salad

8 ounces turkey breast cutlet, cut into 1-inch pieces

1⅔ cups canned white beans, rinsed and drained

4 ounces veggie pepperoni, chopped

¼ cup white wine vinegar

6 ounces canned beets, drained and sliced

Cooking oil spray

1 teaspoon dried oregano

1 teaspoon dried basil

Salt and cracked black pepper to taste

1. Spray a nonstick skillet with cooking spray and heat the skillet. Add the turkey pieces and sear on both sides. Cook about 2 minutes or until they are golden brown.

2. In a mixing bowl, combine the turkey, white beans, veggie pepperoni, vinegar, oregano, basil, salt, and pepper. Toss gently.

To Serve: Arrange the beet slices on plates and spoon the turkey mixture over the beets.

Servings: 2

NOTE: Serve this salad hot or cold.

White Fish and Vegetables en Papillote with Brown Rice

1. Preheat the oven to 325°F. Combine the onion powder, paprika, lemon pepper, red pepper flakes, garlic powder, salt, and cracked black pepper. Sprinkle over the snapper. Cut two sheets of foil larger than the fish fillets in the shape of a heart. Lightly coat the foil with cooking spray. Place a piece of fish on each piece of foil and arrange the carrots and bell pepper around the fish. Drizzle the lemon juice over the fish and vegetables and carefully seal the edges of the foil.

2. Place the packets in a shallow pan with ¼ cup water. Cover the pan and bake for 10 minutes.

To Serve: Place the packets on plates. Snip the top of the foil with scissors and let the steam escape. Serve the fish with the rice. Garnish with lemon wedges, if desired.

Servings: 2

8 ounces boneless snapper fillets

2 cups carrots cut into strips

½ cup red bell pepper cut into thin strips

2 tablespoons freshly squeezed lemon juice

1⅔ cups cooked brown rice

1 tablespoon onion powder

1 teaspoon paprika

1 teaspoon lemon pepper

1 teaspoon red pepper flakes

½ tablespoon garlic powder

Salt and cracked black pepper to taste

Cooking oil spray

Lemon wedges (optional)

Your 5-Week 5-Factor Menu Plan

These menu plans are a great way to start the 5-Factor Diet. All of the foods listed are recipes from this book. Of course, you can always make up your own menus based on the 5-Factor foods you love.

WEEK ONE

DAY 1

Breakfast: Open-Face Egg and Bacon Sandwiches, p. 121

Snack 1: Chocolate-Mint Shakes, p. 180

Lunch: Antipasto, p. 184

Snack 2: Spicy Jumbo Shrimp with Black Bean Dip, p. 156

Dinner: Southern-Style Baked Chicken with Black-Eyed Peas and Collard Greens, p. 226

DAY 2

Breakfast: Oatmeal-Berry Pancakes, p. 131

Snack 1: Hard-Boiled Eggs Stuffed with Tuna Salad, p. 152

Lunch: Green Bean Salad with Tuna and Grapefruit-Scallion Vinaigrette, p. 205

Snack 2: Chicken and Swiss Bites, p. 140

Dinner: Scallop Ratatouille, p. 221

DAY 3

Breakfast: Asparagus Crepes with Toast, p. 112

Snack 1: Apple Wedges with Cinnamon Cream, p. 174

Lunch: Snapper Ceviche with Sweet Potato Rounds, p. 204

Snack 2: Chicken Slices with Cheese and Crackers, p. 145

Dinner: Spaghetti and Meatballs, p. 228

DAY 4

Breakfast: Ham Steaks with Applesauce and Toast, p. 129

Snack 1: Sautéed Peaches with Cheese, p. 175

Lunch: Mushroom-Barley Risotto, p. 196

Snack 2: Hot Dog Skewers with Cherry Tomatoes and Pickles, p. 154

Dinner: Seared Scallops with Orange Sauce and Broccoli-Cauliflower Sauté, p. 223

DAY 5

Breakfast: Smoked Salmon Omelet with Cream Cheese and Whole Grain Toast, p. 126

Snack 1: Roasted Asparagus Spears with Turkey Slices, p. 147

Lunch: Black Bean Gumbo, p. 187

Snack 2: Berry Protein Shakes, p. 183

Dinner: Chicken Ropa Vieja, p. 211

DAY 6

Breakfast: Kashi GoLean with Nonfat Milk, p. 135

Snack 1: Roast Beef with Carrot-Pear Slaw, p. 155

Lunch: Minestrone, p. 194

Snack 2: Apple-Turkey Roll-Ups with Relish and Mustard, p. 136

Dinner: Chiles Rellenos with Brown Rice, p. 212

DAY 7

Cheat Day

WEEK TWO

DAY 1

Breakfast: Bran Pancakes with Ricotta, p. 130

Snack 1: Sautéed Apples over Rice Cakes, p. 163

Lunch: Mixed Greens with Turkey and Cheese Quesadillas, p. 195

Snack 2: Bruschetta, p. 138

Dinner: Warm White Bean, Beet, and Turkey Salad, p. 230

DAY 2

Breakfast: Fully Charged Fruit Salad, p. 133

Snack 1: Belgian Endive Stuffed with Cheesy Artichoke Spread, p. 137

Lunch: Smoked Salmon Pizza, p. 203

Snack 2: Grilled Chicken Kabobs with Carrot-Ginger Vinaigrette, p. 144

Dinner: Salmon with Cucumber-Dill Salad, p. 220

DAY 3

Breakfast: Broccoli-Cheddar Omelet, p. 117

Snack 1: Apple Wedges with Cinnamon Cream, p. 174

Lunch: Chicken and Rice Miso Soup, p. 188

Snack 2: Chips and Salsa, p. 161

Dinner: Creamy Lemon-Ginger Halibut with Corn on the Cob, p. 215

DAY 4

Breakfast: Red Bell Pepper Frittata with Baked Yams, p. 122

Snack 1: Cottage Cheese and Pears, p. 165

Lunch: Greek-Style Shrimp and Spinach Salad, p. 202

Snack 2: Crunchy Celery Sticks with Roasted-Garlic Hummus and Smoked Turkey, p. 142

Dinner: 5-Factor Lasagna, p. 208

DAY 5

Breakfast: Breakfast Burritos I, p. 114

Snack 1: Tropical Berry Protein Shakes, p. 182

Lunch: Baked Potato Skins with Sloppy Joe, p. 186

Snack 2: Gelatin with Berries and Yogurt, p. 176

Dinner: Turkey Fajitas, p. 229

DAY 6

Breakfast: Salmon-Leek Frittata with Whole Grain Toast, p. 123

Snack 1: Toast with Berries and Cocoa Cottage Cheese, p. 168

Lunch: Chicken Fingers and French Fries, p. 189

Snack 2: White Bean Dip, p. 160

Dinner: White Fish and Vegetables en Papillote with Brown Rice, p. 231

DAY 7

Cheat Day

WEEK THREE

DAY 1

Breakfast: French Toast with Ricotta, p. 132

Snack 1: Strawberry-Oatmeal Bars with Yogurt, p. 167

Lunch: Chinese Chicken Wraps with Peanut-Soy Sauce, p. 190

Snack 2: Chocolate-Berry Parfaits, p. 171

Dinner: Seared Halibut with Creamed Spinach and Brown Rice, p. 222

DAY 2

Breakfast: Sweet Potato Home Fries and Scrambled Eggs, p. 128

Snack 1: Fruit Skewers with Cottage Cheese, p. 166

Lunch: Open-Face Turkey BLT, p. 197

Snack 2: Lemon Pie, p. 179

Dinner: Country-Style Ham Steaks with Yams and Corn on the Cob, p. 213

DAY 3

Breakfast: Frittata Italiana, p. 113

Snack 1: Espresso Panna Cotta, p. 172

Lunch: Harley's Sweet Potato Melt, p. 191

Snack 2: Salmon Sashimi with Plums, p. 149

Dinner: Spaghetti and Meatballs, p. 228

DAY 4

Breakfast: Cream of Wheat and Protein, p. 134

Snack 1: Egg Salad with Toast Points, p. 150

Lunch: Baked Chicken and Black Bean Quesadillas with Salsa, p. 185

Snack 2: Fresh Figs with Balsamic Cream Sauce, p. 173

Dinner: Cream of Broccoli Soup with Sauteed Shrimp, p. 214

DAY 5

Breakfast: Scrambled Egg Casserole, p. 124

Snack 1: Chocolate-Mint Shakes, p. 180

Lunch: Pink Pizza, p. 198

Snack 2: Smoked Turkey and Fruit Salad, p. 148

Dinner: Crispy Chicken Tostada, p. 216

DAY 6

Breakfast: Egg and Veggie Muffins, p. 120

Snack 1: Spinach Frittata and Toast, p. 153

Lunch: Salmon Tartare with Arugula, p. 201

Snack 2: Chicken and Swiss Bites, p. 140

Dinner: Bison Steak with Cauliflower-Carrot Mash and Brown Rice, p. 217

DAY 7

Cheat Day

WEEK FOUR

DAY 1

Breakfast: Ham Steaks with Applesauce and Toast., p. 129

Snack 1: Berry Protein Shakes, p. 183

Lunch: Salad Niçoise, p. 200

Snack 2: Egg and Celery Platter with Mustard-Balsamic Sauce, p. 151

Dinner: Indian-Style Chicken with Curried Yogurt Sauce and Brown Rice, p. 218

DAY 2

Breakfast: Oatmeal-Berry Pancakes, p. 131

Snack 1: Apple-Turkey Roll-Ups with Relish and Mustard, p. 136

Lunch: Stuffed Mushrooms and Greens, p. 206

Snack 2: Chicken Salad with Apples, p. 141

Dinner: Lobster and Peas with Tomato-Basil Sauce and Barley, p. 219

DAY 3

Breakfast: Scrambled Eggs with Toast and Grapefruit, p. 125

Snack 1: Raspberry Gelatin with Cottage Cheese, p. 177

Lunch: Mixed Greens with Turkey and Cheese Quesadillas, p. 195

Snack 2: Edamame and Tuna Sashimi with Ginger-Scallion Vinaigrette, p. 143

Dinner: Shrimp and Rice Stir-Fry, p. 225

DAY 4

Breakfast: Breakfast Burritos II, p. 115

Snack 1: Carrot Sticks with Onion Dip, p. 151

Lunch: Antipasto, p. 184

Snack 2: Cheese Course, p. 139

Dinner: Southern-Style Baked Chicken with Black-Eyed Peas and Collard Greens, p. 226

DAY 5

Breakfast: Smoked Turkey and Tomato Scrambled Eggs with Toast, p. 127

Snack 1: Pesto Crisps with Tomatoes and Cheese, p. 162

Lunch: Minestrone, p. 194

Snack 2: Cheesecake, p. 170

Dinner: Salmon with Cucumber-Dill Salad, p. 220

DAY 6

Breakfast: Bell Pepper Pancakes with Mozzarella and Crisp Bacon, p. 118

Snack 1: Pears with Peanut Butter Dip, p. 164

Lunch: Mediterranean-Style Chicken and Quinoa Salad, p. 192

Snack 2: Chips and Salsa, p. 161

Dinner: Chicken Chow Mein, p. 210

DAY 7

Cheat Day

WEEK FIVE

DAY 1

Breakfast: Smoked Salmon Omelet with Cream Cheese and Whole Grain Toast, p. 126

Snack 1: Sauteed Apples over Rice Cakes, p. 163

Lunch: Black Bean Gumbo, p. 187

Snack 2: Crunchy Celery Sticks with Roasted-Garlic Hummus and Smoked Turkey, p. 142

Dinner: 5-Factor Lasagna, p. 208

DAY 2

Breakfast: Open-Face Egg and Bacon Sandwiches, p. 121

Snack 1: Pear and Arugula Salad with Ricotta, p. 146

Lunch: Tuscan Tomato Soup, p. 207

Snack 2: Chicken Slices with Cheese and Crackers, p. 145

Dinner: Argentine-Style Steak Salad with Watercress and Mustard-Cilantro Vinaigrette, p. 209

DAY 3

Breakfast: The Cowboy Omelet, p. 119

Snack 1: Passion Fruit and Tangerine Shakes, p. 181

Lunch: Mexican Chicken Salad with Spicy Salsa Dressing, p. 193

Snack 2: Bruschetta, p. 138

Dinner: Shrimp and Tofu Soup, p. 224

DAY 4

Breakfast: Breakfast Burritos III, p. 116

Snack 1: Toast with Berries and Cocoa Cottage Cheese, p. 168

Lunch: Mixed Greens with Turkey and Cheese Quesadillas, p. 195

Snack 2: Butterscotch and Apple Pudding, p. 169

Dinner: Chicken Ropa Vieja, p. 211

DAY 5

Breakfast: Asparagus Crepes with Toast, p. 112

Snack 1: Grilled Chicken Kabobs with Carrot-Ginger Vinaigrette, p. 144

Lunch: Mushroom Barley Risotto, p. 196

Snack 2: Berry Protein Shakes, p. 183

Dinner: Scallop Ratatouille, p. 221

DAY 6

Breakfast: Broccoli-Cheddar Omelet, p. 117

Snack 1: Fruit Skewers with Cottage Cheese, p. 166

Lunch: Portobello and Turkey Stacks, p. 199

Snack 2: Lemon Yogurt with Kiwi, p. 178

Dinner: Soy-Poached Chicken with Vegetables and Brown Rice, p. 227

DAY 7

Cheat Day

CHAPTER 11

5-Factor Success Log

Writing down what you eat makes you think about your food three times.

First, you think about it as you eat it.

Second, you think about it when you write it down.

Third, you think about it when you read later on.

I've found that thinking three times about everything you eat gives you a sense of ownership of your actions. It also gives you a mini-assessment every day on how well you're doing with your diet. Rome wasn't built in one night. Seeing a few weeks' worth of food logs that show how much better you're eating can be the inspiration you need to stay the course. In fact it's been shown that people who keep track of what they eat are more successful with their nutritional goals.

Still I know you don't have time to write down every calorie and every fat gram from every bite you eat. I wouldn't expect that from my clients, and I don't expect it from you. So here's the good news: You don't have to.

Keeping track of how well you're doing on the 5-Factor Diet isn't painful. It doesn't require a calculator or more than a few seconds of your time.

All of the recipes in this book incorporate 5-Factor Diet requirements—you don't even have to think about them.

When you're ready to create your own meals and daily menus based on the 5-Factor principles—and using the 5-Factor Must-Have Foods—this easy-to-use chart will help you track your progress. (Make copies of it to use every day.)

Record the three foods—a low-fat protein, a low- to moderate-GI carb, and a no- to low-sugar beverage—you plan to eat at each of the five meals of the day. As for the fiber column, if you're eating a low-GI carb, I guarantee it contains the 5 to 10 grams of fiber required at each meal. If necessary, add another fibrous carbohydrate—beans or spinach, for example—to your meal so you can write "yes" in the fiber column. You must have 5 to 10 grams of fiber at every meal to follow the 5-Factor Diet.

The last column, healthy fats, needn't read "yes" at every meal. Just be sure you aren't eating any unhealthy saturated or trans fats.

Ready to start your 5-Factor day? Here you go!

5-FACTOR DIET DAY—SAMPLE

Here's what an average day of eating on the 5-Factor Diet might look like:

Meal	Protein	Low- to moderate-GI carbs	No- to low-sugar beverage	Does it have 5–10 grams of fiber?	Does it have healthy fats? *
Breakfast	3 egg whites	Food for Life's Ezekiel No-Flour Cinnamon Bread toast	Coffee with Splenda	Yes	Yes
Snack 1	Fat-free cheese slice	1-2 apples	Diet soda	Yes	Yes
Lunch	Chicken sandwich w/mustard; side of black beans	Food for Life's Ezekiel No-Flour Tortilla Wrap	Diet Snapple	Yes	Yes
Snack 2	Turkey jerky	Side of steamed veggies	Sugar-free Hansen's	Yes	Yes
Dinner	Steamed salmon	Kashi 7 Whole Grain Pilaf	Green tea	Yes	Yes

*Note: Not every meal must include a healthy fat. For instance, you may choose a low- or no-fat snack that still fits the rest of the 5-Factor criteria. Just be sure that your meal does not include any unhealthy fats (saturated fats or trans fats).

YOUR 5-FACTOR DIET DAY

Meal	Protein	Low- to moderate-GI carbs	No- to low-sugar beverage	Does it have 5–10 grams of fiber?	Does it have healthy fats?*
Breakfast					
Snack I					
Lunch					
Snack 2					
Dinner					

*Note: Not every meal must include a healthy fat. For instance, you may choose a low- or no-fat snack that still fits the rest of the 5-Factor criteria. Just be sure that your meal does not include any unhealthy fats (saturated fats or trans fats).

YOUR 5-FACTOR DIET DAY

Meal	Protein	Low- to moderate-GI carbs	No- to low-sugar beverage	Does it have 5–10 grams of fiber?	Does it have healthy fats?*
Breakfast					
Snack I					
Lunch					
Snack 2					
Dinner					

*Note: Not every meal must include a healthy fat. For instance, you may choose a low- or no-fat snack that still fits the rest of the 5-Factor criteria. Just be sure that your meal does not include any unhealthy fats (saturated fats or trans fats).

YOUR 5-FACTOR WEEKLY PLAN

Once you get used to designing your 5-Factor meals, it's easy to design
your own weekly meal plan, using many of the foods I suggested earlier—
especially the 5-Factor Must-Have Foods.

YOUR 5-FACTOR DIET WEEK

Meal	Breakfast	Snack 1	Lunch	Snack 2	Dinner
Monday					
Tuesday					
Wednesday					
Thursday					
Friday					
Saturday					
Sunday	Cheat Day!				

YOUR 5-FACTOR DIET WEEK

Meal	Breakfast	Snack I	Lunch	Snack 2	Dinner
Monday					
Tuesday					
Wednesday					
Thursday					
Friday					
Saturday					
Sunday	Cheat Day!				

Index

Recipe Index